HIV, Substance Abuse, and Communication Disorders in Children

Haworth Psychosocial Issues of HIV/AIDS
R. Dennis Shelby, PhD
Editor

HIV, Substance Abuse, and Communication Disorders in Children

Robert Martin Screen, PhD
Dorian Lee-Wilkerson, PhD

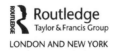

Routledge
Taylor & Francis Group

LONDON AND NEW YORK

Transferred to Digital Printing 2008 by Routledge 2008
2 Park Square, Milton Park, Abingdon, Oxon, OX14 4RN
270 Madison Ave, New York NY 10016

For more information on this book or to order, visit
http://www.haworthpress.com/store/product.asp?sku=5438

or call 1-800-HAWORTH (800-429-6784) in the United States and Canada
or (607) 722-5857 outside the United States and Canada

or contact orders@HaworthPress.com

The Haworth Press, Inc. 10 Alice Street, Binghamton, NY 13904-1580.

PUBLISHER'S NOTE
The development, preparation, and publication of this work has been undertaken with great care. However, the Publisher, employees, editors, and agents of The Haworth Press are not responsible for any errors contained herein or for consequences that may ensue from use of materials or information contained in this work. The Haworth Press is committed to the dissemination of ideas and information according to the highest standards of intellectual freedom and the free exchange of ideas. Statements made and opinions expressed in this publication do not necessarily reflect the views of the Publisher, Directors, management, or staff of The Haworth Press, Inc., or an endorsement by them.

PUBLISHER'S NOTE
Identities and circumstances of individuals discussed in this book have been changed to protect confidentiality.

Cover design by Marylouise E. Doyle.

Library of Congress Cataloging-in-Publication Data

Screen, Robert Martin.
    HIV, substance abuse, and communication disorders in children / Robert Martin Screen, Dorian Lee-Wilkerson.
        p. cm.
    Includes bibliographical references and index.
    ISBN-13: 978-0-7890-2711-5 (case 13 : alk. paper)
    ISBN-10: 0-7890-2711-9 (case 10 : alk. paper)
    ISBN-13: 978-0-7890-2712-2 (soft 13 : alk. paper)
    ISBN-10: 0-7890-2712-7 (soft 10 : alk. paper)
    1. Child development. 2. Children of prenatal substance abuse. 3. Fetus—Effect of drugs on. 4. Communicative disorders in children. I. Lee-Wilkerson, Dorian. II. Title.
    [DNLM: 1. Communication Disorders—etiology. 2. Child. 3. HIV Infections—complications. 4. Prenatal Exposure Delayed Effects. 5. Substance—Related Disorders—complications. WL 340.2 S433h 2007]

RJ520.P74H5822 2007
618.92'869-dc22   2006023763

Publisher's Note
The publisher has gone to great lengths to ensure the quality of this reprint but points out that some imperfections in the original may be apparent.

The authors would like to thank those contributors to the text who provided case study information and Ms. Tracey Weber for her assistance with recruiting these contributors.

CONTENTS

ABOUT THE AUTHORS

Robert Martin Screen, PhD, is chair and professor in the Department of Communicative Sciences and Disorders at Hampton University in Virginia. He has published more than twenty-five articles and is the author of *Multicultural Perspectives in Communication Disorders*. Dr. Screen received the Honors of the Association Award from the American Speech-Language-Hearing Association (ASHA), of which he is a fellow, and he received the Commonwealth of Virginia's Outstanding Faculty Award in 2001.

Dorian Lee-Wilkerson, PhD, is associate professor and director of Graduate Studies in Communicative Sciences and Disorders at Hampton University in Virginia. She specializes in child language disorders and multicultural perspectives in communication disorders.

HIV, Substance Abuse, and Communication Disorders in Children
© 2007 by The Haworth Press, Inc. All rights reserved.
doi:10.1300/5438_a

CONTRIBUTOR

Lemmietta G. McNeilly, PhD, CCC-SLP, ASHA Fellow, is Chief Staff Officer, Speech-Language Pathology of the American Speech-Language-Hearing Association. She received a BS from Hampton Institute, an MA from South Carolina State College, and a doctorate from Howard University.

HIV, Substance Abuse, and Communication Disorders in Children
© 2007 by The Haworth Press, Inc. All rights reserved.
doi:10.1300/5438_b

Foreword

THE NEW ETIOLOGIES

Within the past two decades, there has been an evolution among research studies investigating the etiologies of communication disorders. Today's research on organic and neurogenic communication disorders is exploring etiologies which, prior to the 1960s, were unknown and uninvestigated. Prior to the 1980s, much of our attention and study was focused on communication disorders resulting from systemic congenital and acquired etiologies. Subsequently, during the 1980s and 1990s, medical and clinical research expanded the investigations of consequences that can occur from extrinsic, or environmental, etiologies. Scattered throughout the most recent medical and clinical research literature are studies of the influence of environmental etiologies associated with lifestyle practices. These are, indeed, new etiologies of speech, language, cognitive and developmental disabilities.

This book discusses research that provides the reader with a better understanding of the negative impact that certain maternal lifestyle practices can have upon the child developing in utero and can continue to have upon the young developing child. Specifically, this text presents an analysis of the existing research, which has examined the effects that HIV and maternal substance abuse have upon communication and cognitive development. Additionally, this reference is an acknowledgment of the significant prevalence of HIV and substance abuse in today's society.

This text focuses on the impact of prenatal exposure to drugs, alcohol, and HIV upon young children's development. There has only been scattered attention paid to these issues within the discipline of communication sciences and disorders. This text focuses this scattered research for the benefit of speech-language pathology practitioners and students, and ultimately for the benefit of our clients. The consequences of prenatal exposure to drugs, alcohol, and HIV for the newborn and the developing child can be quite severe. Each chapter in this text provides state-of-the-science research findings and interesting discussions covering pertinent topics such as the neuropathology of drug exposure, as well as the impact of drug exposure, alcohol abuse, and HIV on children's linguistic and cognitive development. The insight gained from these chapters is of critical importance because audiologists and speech-language pathologists are providing clinical services to increasing numbers of children with these new etiology backgrounds.

The knowledge base of our professions is expanding and this text is evidence of the continuing evolution of our clinical research. This text promises to be an important contribution to the professional development of today's communication disorders specialists. This text brings together significant multidisciplinary research on important, newly recognized, etiologies. Children with these etiologies face tremendous developmental and learning challenges and it is the responsibility of professionals to learn as much as they can about these new etiologies and the developmental consequences that many children face because of their mothers' lifestyle practices. As the research frontiers of the twenty-first century expand, new knowledge on other new etiologies will certainly evolve. I am delighted to provide the foreword for a text that is a twenty-first-century trailblazer.

Noma Anderson
Florida International University
Miami, FL;
ASHA Vice President
for Academic Affairs, 1998-2000

Chapter 1

Introduction

In today's ever-changing world, human beings are faced with many dangers. Of these dangers, substance abuse and HIV/AIDS rank extremely high if put into an order, and they can also be fatal if life is not taken seriously. In exploring why this subject is important, one must first take into consideration that these diseases can be life threatening to adults, and to unborn children (in utero). Also, these diseases possess place children into the category of "at risk." Children affected by these diseases may not receive education comparable to that of a "normal" child, or they may simply become victims of arrested development.

This subject is important because substance abuse and HIV/AIDS have been affecting larger populations within recent years, and they can affect the human body in a plethora of ways. However, related to the topic of discussion, these diseases can cause serious difficulties in one's ability to communicate. Also, multicultural populations may be targeted more than others.

Substance abuse includes the misuse of any illegal substances, but for purposes of this discussion, alcohol, marijuana, crack-cocaine, and cocaine will be the focus. Statistically, authors Brown and Toussaint (1997) state that 55,000 infants in the United States are born each year with fetal alcohol syndrome (FAS). Similarly, it is reported that 44 percent of women who drink heavily during pregnancy will have a child with FAS (The National Organization on Fetal Alcohol Syndrome, 1998). Of the other 56 percent, some will have fetal alcohol effects or be exposed to alcohol in utero with minor learning and behavioral difficulties.

HIV, Substance Abuse, and Communication Disorders in Children
© 2007 by The Haworth Press, Inc. All rights reserved.
doi:10.1300/5438_01

Marijuana is the most widely used drug in the United States and research has shown that it has many serious and harmful consequences. Some of the short-term effects include impairments in learning and memory, perception, judgment, and complex motor skills. Thirty-one percent of high school seniors use marijuana today, which is an increase of 40 percent over the past three years. Marijuana use has doubled among eighth graders. Active daily marijuana use is on the rise as well, reaching 3.6 percent among high school seniors in 1994, an increase by 50 percent from that in 1993.

Related to HIV/AIDS, between 800,000 and 1 million Americans are currently infected with HIV. An average of 100 people are diagnosed with AIDS on a daily basis. These alarming numbers indicate how serious the problem of substance abuse and HIV/ AIDS is becoming in our lives today.

Alcohol and drug dependency are increasing every year in our society. As the pressures of everyday life increase, more and more people are turning to alcohol and drugs to escape their pain. The implications of this tragedy are felt far beyond the effects on their users—the impact is extended to their children. Today, there are many children suffering from a variety of disabilities due to in utero. FAS is one such problem.

FAS is defined by Jones et al. (1973), as a pattern of characteristics found in the offspring of alcoholic women. It is a permanent disorder that affects 1 in every 750 live births. As many as 15,000 of the 3 million neonates born in a year will have FAS, with thousands of others exhibiting at least some characteristics of the syndrome (The National Organization on Fetal Alcohol Syndrome, 1998).

These characteristics range from physical and motoric difficulties to mental deficiencies, including emotional and behavioral problems. This syndrome can virtually affect all areas of life. It is also the only disorder that is 100 percent preventable. As a result, steps need to be taken to ensure that women who are alcoholics or heavy drinkers are not allowed to consume alcohol during their pregnancy. Programs need to be developed for the early identification and treatment of children born with FAS.

A review of the literature revealed that there are specific abnormalities in children with FAS. Becker, Warr-Leeper, and Leeper (1990) found that the features and characteristics of FAS include abnormalities of growth, intelligence, behavior, communication, and more. Their study was geared toward the development and deficiencies of children with FAS.

Communication appears to be impaired in all children with FAS, although in varying degrees. Communication can be defined as the use of verbal, gestural, and behavioral skills that allow us to live and participate in social environments. These aspects of communication are greatly altered or impaired in children with FAS.

Deficient cognitive skills are prominent in FAS, although these deficits vary greatly from person to person. Streissguth, Randals, and Smith (1991) found IQs of persons with FAS to be between 30 and 105, which ranges from profound retardation to normal abilities. This range is much broader than what earlier studies from the 1970s and 1980s had found. These studies had a range between 65 and 70, but the size of the samples was small and the population surveyed was limited.

Neurophysiological deficits have been examined for this population using magnetic resonance imaging (MRI) and electroencephalogram (EEG). The results revealed that there are abnormalities in the corpus callosum, and reduced volume of several subcortical brain structures that are not believed to be the result of microcephaly.

The degree of intellectual impairment has been found to be associated with the severity of the physical anomalies of those with FAS/FAE. Therefore, the more physical involvement the person has, the greater the cognitive impairment, and the less physical involvement the higher the cognitive skills.

Regardless of the person's IQ, those with FAS/FAE exhibit extreme difficulty with mathematical computations and reasoning/problem-solving tasks. These problems persist into adulthood and are the precipitating reasons why many of those with FAS are unable to live independently as adults (Streissguth, Randals, and Smith, 1991).

IMPORTANCE TO COMMUNICATION DISORDERS

As stated previously, these syndromes possess the ability to cause serious harm to one's ability to communicate. For example, some symptoms that may be acquired involve swollen glands. Speech impairment is a symptom that may be present when diagnosed with

HIV/AIDS. Neurological signs are present in 10 to 20 percent of HIV patients when first diagnosed. Fifty to seventy percent will develop AIDS dementia or AIDS-related cognitive-motor complex, which are characteristic patterns of cognitive, motor, and behavioral dysfunctions. Also, 60 to 90 percent of AIDS patients show some form of pathology to the brain at autopsy. The virus enters the brain, localizes itself in the central nervous system (CNS), and spreads throughout the brain. AIDS causes neurologic manifestations occurring in the ear, nose, and throat that unfortunately interfere with communication; neurologic disease is identifiable in the form of opportunistic infections and tumors as well as peripheral neuropaths. Patients with dementia have difficulty, and slowing, of speech. About 50 percent of all AIDS patients are affected by ear, nose, and throat complications. Of these, the most common complication of the ear is Kaposi's sarcoma of the external ear (a malignant tumor). In addition, possible problems related to communication disorders are as follows: oral candidasis (a fungal infection caused by yeast), herpes simplex virus infection (recurrent inflammatory virus disease affecting the mouth, lips, or face), hairy leukoplakia (thick, white patches covering the tongue, gums, etc.), gingivitis (inflammation of the gums) and periodontal disease (disease occurring around the teeth), and aphthous ulcers (white spots/pustules caused by viral or fungal infections).

MINORITY POPULATIONS

One in 250 people in the United States is infected with human immunodeficiency virus (HIV), which causes AIDS, and it is the leading cause of death among men and women between the ages of twenty-five and forty-four. Age and development stages, early initiation of sexual behaviors, sexual identifiers, self-esteem, untreated sexually transmitted diseases (STDs), and the use of alcohol and other drugs are considered to be contextual influences that increase the risk of AIDS. Data related to this topic indicate that the infection rate is increasing among African-American, Latino, and younger homosexual men. Intravenous (IV) drug users are at risk because of unavailability of sterile injection equipment and use of infected needles. Since the 1990s, women of color have increased drastically as a risk group in the United States and constitute 50 percent of the infections worldwide. Much of this increase can be attributed to choosing sexual partners who are drug users. Also, vertical transmission from infected mother to infant continues to be a source of high risk for infants (U.S. Department of Health and Human Services, 1998).

African-American and Hispanic communities are being hit extremely hard by this epidemic. African Americans make up 28 percent of all diagnosed AIDS cases and Hispanics make up 16 percent; of these cases attributed to IV drug use, African Americans account for 45 percent of the cases and Hispanics account for 26 percent. Substance abuse enhances the spread of HIV infection through sharing of needles and the practice of unsafe sex related to the use of crack, alcohol, and other substances.

The rate of HIV infection is growing at a high rate among minorities. Data indicate that 30 to 40 percent of all Americans with HIV are minorities. The rate of HIV transmission is spreading most rapidly in women and children. Of all women with AIDS, 76 percent are women of color and of all the children, 82 percent are minority children. Racial and ethnic minority populations have been disproportionately affected by HIV infection and AIDS since the beginning of the epidemic in the United States. Through June 1993, the Centers for Disease Control and Prevention (CDC) reported 315,390 cases of AIDS in the United States, including 97,794 cases among blacks, 52,531 among Hispanics, 2,036 among Asians/Pacific Islanders, and 657 among American Indians/Alaskan Native. Through mid-1993, 48 percent of all reported AIDS cases were among blacks and Hispanics. However, these two population groups represent only 21 percent of the total U.S. population. In 1991, HIV/AIDS was the sixth leading cause of death among Hispanics, while it ranked tenth among whites. Both the proportions of deaths and the death rates associated with HIV/AIDS are substantially higher for black and Hispanic women than for women in other racial/ethnic populations.

According to an ASHA report on communication disorders and HIV, 50 percent of all male heterosexual HIV cases are reportedly African Americans. Another statistic in the ASHA report revealed that, through a research study in an urban community, one out of forty African-American and Hispanic-American twenty-one-year-old Job Corps applicants tested positive for HIV. Five years later, the same urban community was tested and the calculations were five times greater (ASHA, 1997).

The spread of HIV among young women is greater in urban communities. The states with the highest female death rates due to HIV and AIDS are Washington, DC, New Jersey, New York, Florida, Connecticut, Delaware, and Maryland. These same states also have high urban community population.

Persons with AIDS may experience problems related to hearing, comprehension, conveying messages to others, speech problems (i.e., loudness, rate, speech–sound differentiation), language problems, and aphasia (i.e., dementia). Other problems that affect persons with AIDS may be interferences such as endotracheal intubation and tracheotomy.

An entirely new area of research has opened now for specialists in communication disorders. The problem encountered by schoolchildren who are victims of the abuse that occurs from the use of illegal substances and from HIV infection are problems must be studied.

This book, we hope, is the beginning of many more such discussions on these problems. We anticipate an outpouring of research interest and direction, which will provide us the information that is so desperately needed.

REFERENCES

ASHA (1997). Communication Disorders and HIV: The HIV Treatment Community's Guide to Working with Speech-Language Pathologists. Author.

Becker, M., Warr-Leeper, G.A., and H.A. Leeper (1990). Fetal Alcohol Syndrome: A Description of Oral Motor, Articulatory, Short Term Memory, Grammatical, and Semantic Abilities. *Journal of Communication Disorders.* April; 23 (2), 97-124.

Brown, D. and P. Toussaint (1997). *The Black Woman's Guide to Pregnancy, Childbirth, and Baby's First Year.* New York: Dutton.

Jones, K., Smith, D. et al. (1973). Recognition of the Fetal Alcohol Syndrome in Early Infancy. *Lancet.* 999-1001.

The National Organization on Fetal Alcohol Syndrome (Fetal Alcohol Syndrome Prevention) (1998). Washington, DC: Author.

Streissguth, A. (1997). *Fetal Alcohol Syndrome: A Guide for Families and Communities.* Paul H. Brookes Publishing Co. 9-35.

Streissguth, A., Randels, S., and D. Smith (1991). Test-Retest Study of Intelligence in Patients with Fetal Alcohol Syndrome: Implications for Care. *The Journal of the American Academy of Child and Adolescent Psychiatry.* 30 (4), 584-587.

United States Department of Health and Human Services (Fetal Alcohol Syndrome Prevention) (1998). Rockville, MD: Author.

Chapter 2

The Nature of Substance Abuse and Language Disorders

Twenty years ago, it would have been difficult to imagine that the future would present an explosion in the population of children and adults with communicative disorders as a result of substance abuse that has pervaded our society in more recent years. Due to the complexity of our society, its growing pains, its pressures, and the inability to "cope," which is all too prevalent, more and more persons have turned to substances. Myriad reasons exist for this, indeed, that could explain why this has happened, and it could be the subject of an entire course of study. Nevertheless, the fact remains that substance abuse during pregnancy is on the rise, and we are even more aware of its effect on the children, who are prenatally exposed to drugs.

This chapter discusses the nature of this problem and looks at specific drugs and how they impact upon communication disorders.

PREVALENCE

Today, the use/abuse of tobacco, alcohol, and illicit drugs is a societal variable that must be considered when one attempts to identify, describe, and treat a communicative disorder. One can speculate that tobacco, alcohol, and illicit drugs are used by more of the world's total population because they are more accessible today than ever before. Also, social acceptance justifies and validates the use of these substances.

HIV, Substance Abuse, and Communication Disorders in Children
© 2007 by The Haworth Press, Inc. All rights reserved.
doi:10.1300/5438_02

Although the estimates of prevalence vary, some have estimated that one-half to three-quarters of a million infants are born each year with in-utero exposure to illicit drugs. When tobacco and alcohol are added, the figures rise to more than 1 million exposed infants (Brady et al., 1994).

Recent state surveys have shown that between 8 and 12 percent of women giving birth in hospitals had used illegal drugs sometime during the pregnancy, including just before delivery (Statewide Prevalence of Illicit Drug Use by Pregnant Women, 1990; Vega et al., 1993). These studies support information from a study in Pinellas County, Florida, which demonstrated that illicit substance use during pregnancy occurs across all racial and socioeconomic lines (Chasnoff, Landress, and Barrett, 1990). In addition to the use of illegal drugs, the use of alcohol before delivery is also identified as a problem (Nalty, 1991).

Chasnoff and Griffith (1989) estimate that 11 percent of all newborns, more than 459,690 children, each year are exposed to illicit drugs. Gomby and Shiono (1991) estimate that more than 739,000 women each year use one or more illegal substances during pregnancy. The effect that prenatal drug exposure has on a child's language development, among other things, is especially devastating.

LANGUAGE DELAYS

One of the most frequently reported characteristics of children with prenatal drug exposure is poor language development. Some children acquire speech late, while others speak infrequently (Cohen and Taharally, 1992). Identifying language delays not only involves targeting children who present with language problems. Research is being conducted to identify variables that put children in jeopardy of developing language problems. One variable that is being studied is prenatal drug exposure (Reed, 1994).

Several long-term studies have demonstrated that substance-exposed infants are at risk of acquiring developmental and learning problems. A range of language and speech delays, including language-processing problems, poor articulation, limited vocabulary, and limited expressive language skills, are among current findings. Some children do not understand a simple question such as, "Are you hungry?" Even at five years of age, some are unable to follow two-step commands. Another characteristic of these children's language-processing problem is their inability to understand the real meaning of words and to generalize these "symbols of experience" to new similar situations. A typical example is as follows: if you tell a child not to go into the street, he or she does not understand that you mean all streets (Brady et al., 1994).

Many practitioners identified poor articulation as a common problem, which makes children's communication attempts unintelligible to both teachers and peers. The superintendent (Dr. Charlie Knight) at the Parent-Child Intervention Program (PCIP) in East Palo Alto, Texas, reported that some of the children could not enunciate the word "potty" well enough to make themselves understood, thus resulting in a large number of toileting mishaps (Brady et al., 1994).

The children's inability to make their needs known and their lack of vocabulary are likely to cause them to behave aggressively and to be disruptive during class. Their limited language skills inhibit their ability to engage in imaginative play. "Taking on a role and acting it out are crucial to developing more advanced forms of play" (Brady et al., 1994). The following is an example of one disruptive child:

> One little girl was very distant with the teachers in the classroom. She was aggressive with the other children and would strike out and hit them. As we worked with her, especially on her expressive language skills, her behavior started to improve. She was finally able to express her needs and feelings. It is hard to know exactly why she had no communication skills. Perhaps it was related to her exposure to drugs prenatally. (Brady et al., 1994)

Speech and language problems are one of the behaviors that is troubling professionals working with children who have been prenatally exposed to drugs. These problems can hinder such things as learning and social development. Practitioners are just beginning to look into the cohort of children, in kindergarten and in the primary grades, who were prenatally exposed to drugs and other risks. If such problems persist, children will be at risk of experiencing failure in school (Brady et al., 1994).

Children who are in the first through third grades are in the early stages of learning to write and read. Children who are prenatally exposed to drugs will have severe problems with this stage in their school career. According to Brady et al. (1994), language is both the curriculum content and the learning environment, both the object of knowledge and the medium through which knowledge is acquired.

The complicity of substance abuse carries with it serious social issues, such as crime, domestic violence, and traffic injuries. However, the devastating role that substance abuse plays in communication is an issue just recently discovered by those in the research field. We now examine the most commonly used/abused substances and provide a brief description of the impact these substances have upon communication disorders.

TOBACCO

The risk associated with cigarette smoking during pregnancy has been well documented. Despite the known consequences many expectant mothers continue to smoke cigarettes. The Center for Disease Control and Prevention/National Center for Health Statistics reports that 17 percent of women report having smoked during pregnancy (Ventura et al., 1994). Women who smoke cigarettes while pregnant tend to be younger, poorer, and less educated (Fried, 1992). Studies of effects of tobacco show that auditory responsiveness, with infants less than a week of age, was altered among babies born to women who smoked while pregnant (Fried et al., 1992).

Studies conducted on children prenatally exposed to tobacco also suggest that deficits linked to maternal smoking during pregnancy are not conquered by three years of age. The cognitive functioning of three-year-old children born to mothers who smoked ten or more cigarettes a day during pregnancy showed a lower level of performance compared to children of mothers who quit smoking while pregnant on the McCarthy Scales of Children's Abilities and the Minnesota Child Development Inventory (McCance-Katz, 1991).

In a string of longitudinal studies, children up to the age of eleven, who were exposed prenatally to cigarette smoke, show diminished ability in auditory processing and language/verbal competence (Kindlon and Feton, 1994). Sexton et al. (1990) have found small differences in the general cognitive ability between exposed and nonexposed children. Fried and colleagues (1992) have found an association between prenatal cigarette exposure and both impulsive behavior and impaired memory in six-year-olds.

Cigarette smoking also affects the cognitive processes among adult smokers. Among the adult population cigarette smoking is a relatively common occurrence; in the United States alone, approximately 54 million adults smoke (Spilich et al., 1992). Many smokers believe that smoking helps them to think and concentrate.

Spilich et al. (1992) found no deviations related to cigarette smoking in tasks that require low to moderate effort, that are high in automaticity, and place no demand on the long-term memory.

Further results indicated that cigarettes caused a negative effect upon short-term memory. In addition, this negative effect is maintained among smokers for some time following the termination of smoking (Spilich et al., 1992).

Spilich et al. (1992) concluded that smoking cigarettes is linked to poorer recall and a decreased ability to differentiate critical items of lesser importance. The researchers suggested that disturbances in working memory or attentional capacity, which are involved in dealing with complex tasks, are related to the agents in cigarettes, nicotine, and/or carboxyhemoglobin.

Overall, no conclusion can be made from the Spilich study as to whether cigarette smoking has a positive or negative effect on cognitive performance. More research needs to be conducted before inferences can be drawn.

ALCOHOL

Twenty percent of mothers have reported using alcohol at some point during their pregnancy (Ventura et al., 1994).

Research has found that children prenatally exposed to alcohol can exhibit such problems ranging from full-blown FAS characterized by growth deficits, mental retardation, and behavioral difficulties, to exhibiting only some of these characteristics.

FAS is characterized by pre- or postnatal growth retardation, CNS dysfunction (most commonly) developmental delay, or intellectual impairment and craniofacial abnormalities (Streissguth, 1994). Hyperkinetic and attention problems are most common, and estimates of prevalence are over 70 percent. Conduct disorder is seen in approximately 20 percent of children with FAS (Steinhausen et al., 1993). Elementary schoolchildren with FAS often are hyperactive, distracted easily, and are impulsive and prone to memory difficulties. They lack social skills. As adolescents, they have limited reasoning and judgment abilities and may act impulsively. They also have an ability to think abstractly (Schroeder, 1996).

Very low levels of alcohol appear to have some negative effect on the IQ in early childhood (Jacobson and Jacobson, 1994). This is especially troubling considering that some research has suggested that postnatal environment does not appear to be associated with changes in IQ over time in exposed children (Streissguth, 1994). Streissguth et al. (1989) found a significant negative relationship between alcohol consumption during pregnancy by white, middle-class women and the IQ scores of their offspring at four years of age.

In alcoholic women, it is difficult to isolate the effects of alcohol exposure from those associated with other drugs and social risks. There is also some concern about the accuracy of recall regarding the quantity of alcohol and the frequency of use by the mother (Day, 1992).

According to Tarter et al. (1995), the cognitive capacity of adolescent substance abusers is lower in the following domains: verbal and nonverbal intellectual capacity, perceptual speed, sustained attention, language competence, and academic achievement. The researchers stated that the substance-abused individuals are more impulsive because they are less capable of suppressing motor responses to irrelevant stimuli. The results of their study indicated that the substance abusers demonstrated deficits on six of seven measures of language capacity. In addition, their IQ scores in tests of academic achievement and language competence were lower. Overall, the impulsivity of these individuals is a result of their incapacity to use language effectively.

COCAINE

"Cocaine, once thought to be a harmless recreational drug, now has been shown to have serious effects on infants exposed in utero" (Edelstein, Kropenske, and Howard, 1990). According to Corwin et al. (1992), the cries of infants are affected by in-utero cocaine exposure. The result of their study revealed that the following characterized the cries of the infants: fewer cries, more short cries, they possessed less cries in the hyperphonation mode and also had a higher median fundamental frequency for the first cry utterance. Corwin et al. stated that cocaine-exposed infants generally exhibit tremors, abnormal sucking patterns, and patterns of irritability and unusual cry patterns.

Infants exposed prenatally to crack-cocaine were frequently perceived as fragile and disoriented by their caregivers. They appear to have a low threshold for overstimulation and are unresponsive to social stimulation.

> Many children exposed to crack-cocaine in utero or during their early years have entered the public school programs. A range of behaviors have been observed: irritability, agitation, hyperactivity, speech and language delays, motor delays, poor task organization, processing deficits, poor pragmatic/social skills and short attention spans. (Power-Culver, 1992)

The expected profound cognitive deficits in young children with intrauterine exposure to cocaine have not been seen (Griffith, Azuma, and Chasnoff, 1994; Zuckerman and Frank, 1994). Some studies (Struther and Hanson, 1992) have noted specific cognitive effects but when overall IQ is calculated for children up to three years of age the scores for the exposed children are almost equal to those for the matched nonexposed control group (Kindlon and Feton, 1994).

However, these findings should be taken lightly since the exposed children have not reached school age, and work in other areas (i.e., fetal alcohol exposure) suggests that deficits may not emerge until years later (Griffith, Azuma, and Chasnoff, 1994).

It has been proven to be difficult to isolate the problems seen in infants with prenatal exposure to cocaine to the effects of cocaine alone (Kindlon and Feton, 1994). Many factors known to produce negative outcomes that can be correlated strongly to maternal cocaine use. For instance, expectant mothers who use cocaine tend not to seek prenatal care (Valencia et al., 1989). Also, cocaine is rarely used in isolation, and women who use cocaine also tend to use more alcohol than expectant mothers whose substance use is limited to alcohol (Jacobson and Chiodo, 1996).

Nevertheless, the impact of prenatal crack-cocaine exposure on speech and language skills needs to be studied. At the present time, speech–language pathologists and audiologists will need to interpret information gathered from the research of their colleagues in medicine and psychology (Power-Culver, 1992).

MARIJUANA

Prenatal marijuana use does not seem to affect cognitive or language development in five- to six-year-old children. However, there is very limited data available on the relationship between cognitive performance in young children and prenatal use of marijuana. "At 2 and 3 years of age, after controlling for potential confounding variables, marijuana use during pregnancy was not associated with decreases in cognitive scores. At 4 years, however, significantly lower scores in verbal and memory domains were associated with maternal marijuana use after adjusting for confounding variables" (Fried et al., 1992).

Long-term outcome studies of cannabis-exposed children are not available, but this is clearly an area for further research (McCance-Katz, 1991).

HEROIN

Studies have shown that children who are prenatally exposed to heroin suffer from below-average weight and length, adjustment problems, psycholinguistic and other ability deficits through six years of age.

Furthermore, studies have indicated that infants of heroin-addicted women exhibit a number of behavioral disturbances in early life.

The lasting cognitive-developmental differences between these children and the controls have not consistently been found (Brady et al., 1994).

PHENYLCYCLINDINE HYDROCHLORIDE (PCP)

According to the Los Angeles Department of Health, PCP is second only to hallucinogens in cases of drug overdose. Studies have indicated that children exposed to PCP demonstrate the following: tremors, increase in sensitivity to touch and environmental sounds, increased muscle tone, and abnormal eye movements. These newborns are typically irritable and hypertonic. Van Dyke and Fox (1990) found that infants at nine months of age exhibited gross motor and personal/social skills that were age appropriate. These infants also demonstrated fine motor abilities that appeared to interfere with normal developmental or adaptive behavior. After testing these children later at eighteen and twenty-four months of age, the results indicated that they were below normal in fine motor abilities and in language. Overall, there seems to be a limited amount of information on PCP and its effects on language development.

Combination of Cocaine, Heroin, and Methodone

Infants born to narcotic-dependent mothers exhibit impairment in their interactive ability and may be difficult to engage or console. They tend to be irritable and tremulous with unpredictable behavior (McCance-Katz, 1991).

A longitudinal study conducted by Baar and Graff (1994) found that mothers who used a combination of cocaine, heroin, and methadone during pregnancy had children who showed delays in cognitive functioning at preschool age. Over time, the individual difficulties and differences in developmental patterns were most prominent when language development formed part of the assessments. "Intervention programs should focus on improvements of early language development and communication, in addition to the children's ability to adapt to task situation" (Baar and Graff, 1994).

SUMMARY

Infants of drug-dependent mothers are at risk of acquiring developmental problems, including in the area of language. The precise consequences of prenatal drug exposure are not at all clear, since street drugs such as heroin or cocaine are not pure, but mixed with other substances. Also, there is much variation in the frequency of use and the quantity of drugs taken.

An important factor to consider in successfully evaluating intellectual and language problems of exposed children is whether or not the child was raised in a drug-free or drug-using environment. "Children are much more likely to display problems in verbal reasoning if they were raised in a home where drugs were continued to be used" (Griffith, Azuma, and Chasnoff, 1994). Lack of prenatal care, poor postnatal nutrition, and poor medical care must also be considered.

Also, not all substance-exposed children suffer the same prognosis. Generalizations about drug-exposed children and the effects that this exposure has on language needs additional research before the fate of these children can be known.

One thing that is certain about children prenatally exposed to drugs is that this population does not represent a change in direction. Rather, it presents an increased demand for urgent and detailed research.

REFERENCES

Baar, A. and B. Graff (1994). Cognitive Development at Preschool-Age of Infants of Drug-Dependent Mothers. *Developmental Medicine and Children Neurology.* 36, 383-391.

Brady, Joanne, Posner, Marc, Lang, Cynthia, and Michael Rosati (1994). Risk and Reality: The Implications of Prenatal Exposure to Alcohol and Other Drugs [Online]. Available: Infoseek.

Chasnoff, I.J., Burns, W.J., Schnoll, S.H., and K.A. Burns (1991). Cocaine Use in Pregnancy. *The New England Journal of Medicine.* 313 (11), 666-669.

Chasnoff, I.J. and D.R. Griffith (1989). Temporal Patterns of Cocaine Use in Pregnancy: Adverse Perinatal Outcome. *JAMA.* 313, 666-669.

Chasnoff, I.J., Landress, H., and M. Barrett (1990). The Prevalence of Illicit Drug or Alcohol Use During Pregnancy and Discrepancies in Reporting in Pinellas County, Florida. *New England Journal of Medicine.* 322, 1202-1206.

Cohen, S. and C. Taharally (1992). Getting Ready for Young Children with Prenatal Drug Exposure. *Childhood Education.* Fall Issue.

Corwin et al. (1992). Cocaine Exposed Infants. *Pediatrics.* 89, 1199-1203.

Day, N.L. (1992). The Effects of Prenatal Exposure to Alcohol. *Alcohol Health & Research World.* 16(3), 238-243.

Edelstein, S., Kropenske, V., and J. Howard (1990). Projects T.E.A.M.S. *Social Work.* 35, 313-318.

Fried, P.A. (1992). Marijuana Use by Pregnant Women: Neurobehavioral Effects in Neonates. *Drug Alcohol Depend.* 6, 415-424.

Fried et al. (1992). 60-and 72-Month Follow-Up of Children Prenatally Exposed to Marijuana, Cigarettes and Alcohol: Cognitive and Language Assessment. *Journal of Development and Behavioral Pediatrics.* 13, 383-391.

Gomby and Shiono (1991). Estimating the Number of Substance-Exposed Infants. *Future Child.* 1, 17-25.

Griffith, A., Azuma, S.D., and I.J. Chasnoff (1994). Three-Year Outcome of Children Prenatally Exposed to Drugs. *Journal of the American Academy of Child and Adolescent Psychiatry.* 33, 20-27.

Jacobson and Chiodo (1996). Effects of Heavy Prenatal Cocaine Exposure on Infant Cognition, Paper Presented at the International Conference on Infant Studies. Providence, RI, April 19, 1996.

Jacobson and Jacobson (1994). Prenatal Alcohol Exposure and Neurobehavioral Development: Where Is the Threshold? *Alcohol, Health and Research World.* 18, 30-36.

Kindlon, D.J. and E.R. Feton (1994). The Effects of Prenatal Exposure to Tobacco, Alcohol and Cocaine [Online]. Available: Infoseek.

McCanze-Katz, E. (1991). *Psychosomatics.* 32, 268-273.

Nalty, D.F. (1991). South Carolina Prevalence Study of Drug Use Among Women Giving Birth. Columbia, SC: South Carolina Commission on Alcohol and Drug Abuse.

Power-Culver (1992). Crack-Exposed Babies: Are You Ready for Them? *Education Week.* 23-33.

Reed, V.V. (1994). *An Introduction to Children with Language Disorder.* Second Edition. McMillan Coll. Pub., NY. 157, 163, 41, 44.

Schroeder (1996). Fetal Alcohol Syndrome. *The Education Digest.* 73-75.

Sexton, M. (1990). Prenatal Exposure to Tobacco. *Int. J. Epidemol.* 19, 72-77.

Spilich et al. (1992). Cigarette Smoking and Cognitive Performance. *British Journal of Addiction.* 87, 113-126. [Online]. Available: http://www.washcoll.edu/wc.html/academics/Spilich/2A.html.

Statewide Prevalence of Illicit Drug Use by Pregnant Women-Rhode Island (1990). *MMWR.* 39, 225-227.

Steinhausen et al. (1993). Long-Term Psychopathological and Cognitive Outcome of Children with Fetal Alcohol Syndrome. *Journal of the American of Child and Adolescent Psychiatry.* 32, 990-994.

Streissguth, A.P. (1994). Drinking During Pregnancy Decreases Word Attack and Arithmetic Scores on Standardized Tests. *Alcoholism: Clinical and Experimental Research.* 18, 248-254.

Streissguth et al. (1989). Fetal Alcohol Syndrome in Adolescents and Adults. *Journal of the American Medical Association.* 265, 1961-1967.

Struther and Hanson (1992). Visual Recognition Memory in Drug-Exposed Infants. *Developmental and Behavioral Pediatrics.* 13, 108-111.

Tarter et al. (1995). Drug and Alcohol Dependence. *Journal of Learning Disabilities.* 39, 15-21.

Valencia et al. (1989). Epidemiology of Cocaine Use During Pregnancy at Kings County Hospital Center. *Pediatric Research.* 25, 265A.

Van Dyke and Fox (1990). Fetal Drug Exposure and Its Possible Implications to Learning on Preschool and School-Age Population. *Journal of Learning Disabilities.* 23, 160-165.

Vega W.A., Kolody, B., Hwang, J., and A. Noble (1993). Prevalence and Magnitude of Perinatal Substance Exposure in California. *New England Journal of Medicine.* 329, 850-854.

Ventura, S.J., Martin, A.M., Taffel, S.M., Matthews, T.J., and S.C. Clarke (1994). Advance Report of Final Natality Statistics. *Monthly Vital Statistics Report.* 43.

Zuckerman and Frank (1994). Prenatal Cocaine Exposure: Nine Years Later. *The Journal of Pediatrics.* 124, 731-733.

Chapter 3

The Effects of Drugs on the Brain

SUBSTANCES AND THE BRAIN

We have all seen the commercial, "This is your brain. This is your brain on drugs. Any questions?" However, despite this commercial and other "Just Say No" advertisements, drug abuse is still very prevalent. As speech–language pathologists, we must be aware of the profound effect that drugs such as alcohol, cocaine, and marijuana have on the brain.

The brain is a chemical organ of the body. It contains billions of neurons (brain cells) that connect with each other to form neuron networks. These networks carry all of the functions of thinking, feeling, movement, as well as the senses of the human body. Each neuron is fired by a chemical reaction at the beginning of the cell. The electrical impulse moves through the cell as a result of the chemical reaction. The information from one brain cell (neuron) is carried to the next brain cell across a gap by small packets of chemicals, called neurotransmitters. All mood-altering drugs affect the process of chemical transmission in neuron networks. As drug and alcohol use become regular and more abused, the chemistry of the brain is increasingly distorted.

Alcohol is the most widely used and abused drug in the United States (Bernstein and Tiegerman, 1989). Research shows that alcohol adversely affects the brain. Structural changes in the brains of alcoholics have been reported (Ron, 1979; Wilkinson, 1987), as well as reduced cerebral blood flow and altered electrical activity (Porjesz and Begleiter, 1981).

HIV, Substance Abuse, and Communication Disorders in Children
© 2007 by The Haworth Press, Inc. All rights reserved.
doi:10.1300/5438_03

Tarter and Edwards (1986) summarize evidence suggesting that neuropsychological impairments in alcoholics may occur for a number of reasons. The toxic effects of alcohol on the brain may cause impairment directly. In addition, some alcoholics may exhibit impairment as an indirect result of alcohol abuse; e.g., they may have experienced a craniocerebral trauma or they may be suffering nutritional deficits (such as thiamine or niacin deficiencies).

Cocaine is another drug that can affect the brain. There is no difference between cocaine and "crack" cocaine. Crack is created by mixing the cocaine with water and bicarbonate soda to form a hard substance. The substance allows the cocaine to vaporize. The vaporized cocaine produces a rapid "high" when inhaled. In discussing the effects of cocaine on the brain, it is important to introduce two concepts that are crucial in understanding the reinforcing and addicting properties of cocaine. The first is its ability to block the reuptake of dopamine from the synapse; the second is the presence in the brain of several dopaminergic systems with different behavioral and adaptive properties. The ability of cocaine to inhibit neurotransmitter reuptake has been closely linked to its behavioral actions. Cocaine inhibits the reuptake of dopamine, norepinephrine, and serotonin with equal potency, but many of its behavioral and reinforcing effects appear to result from dopamine reuptake blockade (Wise, 1984). Other effects of cocaine on the CNS include increased respiratory and heart rates, restlessness and excitement (Bernstein and Tiegerman, 1989).

Another drug that also profoundly affects the brain is marijuana. Long-term use of marijuana produces changes in the brain that are similar to those seen after long-term use of other major drugs abuse such as cocaine and alcohol.

Marijuana is a green, brown, or gray mixture of dried, shredded flowers and leaves of the hemp plant *(Cannabis sativa).* Cannabis is a term that refers to marijuana and other drugs made from the same plant. All forms of cannabis are mind-altering (psychoactive) drugs; they all contain THC (delta-9-tetrahydrocannabinol), the main active chemical in marijuana. There are about 400 chemicals in a cannabis plant, but THC is the one that affects the brain the most (U.S. Department of Health and Human Services, 1995).

It has been shown that marijuana smoking affects the brain and leads to impaired short-term memory, perception, judgment, and motor skills. According to the National Institute on Drug Abuse, THC disrupts the nerve cells in the part of the brain where memories are formed. This makes it hard for the user to recall events (such as what happened a few minutes ago), and so it is hard to learn while being "high."

Some studies show that when people have smoked large amounts of marijuana for many years, the drug takes its toll on mental functions. Among a group of longtime heavy marijuana users in Costa Rica, researchers found that the people had great trouble when asked to recall a short list of words (a standard test of memory). People in that study group also found it very hard to focus their attention on the tests given to them (U.S. Department of Health and Human Services, 1995).

Alcohol is a drug that is viewed as "harmless as long as it is consumed within moderation." However, researchers have found in certain studies that even small amounts of alcohol can have negative effects on the brain. Researchers show that a person who drinks alcohol may experience cognitive difficulties, such as impaired memory or reasoning ability. Alcoholics receiving treatment may also have deficits in problem solving, abstract thinking, concept shifting, and psychomotor performance. The amount of alcohol consumed and its relationship to which cognition is impaired has long been researched. Some findings indicate a decrease in test scores among self-reported drinkers (Oscar-Breman, 1992).

The effects of alcohol have often been compared to elderly traits. Researchers explain its effect as premature aging because it often resembles deficits observed in normal elderly persons. Some individuals are considered at risk for alcoholism. One example would be children of alcoholics. Test results indicate that this group may be less adept at certain learning and visual–spatial integration. One recent study discussed by Dr. Steven Chatoff, the medical director of the Exodus Recovery Center in Marina Del Ray, California, show that up to 92 percent of cocaine addicts have a positive family history for alcoholism, drug addiction, or related disorder. He feels this validates the role of genetics, not just in alcohol, but in all drug addictions.

There are two disorders commonly associated with alcoholism. The first is Alcohol Amnestic Disorder (commonly called Korsakoff's Psychosis or Werncke's Korsakoff Syndrome). Two major characteristics of this disorder are short-term memory impairments and behavior changes. The other disorder is dementia. This disorder is typically characterized by global loss of intellectual ability, memory impairment, disturbance in abstract thinking and distorted judgment, and personality change without clouding of consciousness.

Alcohol can also affect the fetus of an expectant mother. What happens when alcohol is consumed by a pregnant mother? Alcohol abuse during pregnancy is related to a series of congenital malformations described as FAS. The characteristics of FAS include a number of severe birth defects.

There is a larger body of research that reports that FAS infants tend to be tremulous, overreactive to sound, have feeding difficulties, irritable, and possess a slow, weak sucking ability. In maturing children, the legacy of material drinking may become evident in tests that indicate marginal mental retardation, short memory span, distractibility, interrupted or unusual sleep patterns, and emotional instability. Later in life these children may be hyperactive, inattentive, impulsive, fearless, and indiscriminate in their reaction to friends and strangers. They also demonstrate poor motor function or thinking disorder (Wilkinson, 1987).

Common physical and behavior denominators shared by this study group included the following:

1. Majority were unusual in regard to head shape, fingers, nose, ears, palms, back/neck/spine/and mid-face
2. Eighty percent had teeth problems
3. Eighty percent experienced neglect
4. Fifty-two percent were victims of child abuse
5. Eighty percent are afflicted with an attention deficit disorder and could not concentrate on a single task for an extended period of time
6. Seventy-three percent had memory problems
7. Seventy-two percent were hyperactive at some point in their development
8. Majority of this population is characterized by willful or inadvertent disobedience or school truancy
9. Ninety-five percent could not handle money on their own regardless of sex, age, or educational level
10. Fifty percent could not care for all their hygienic needs

From the aforementioned results, it is evident that alcohol can have lasting effects on the brain and the development of a fetus, and for some FAS children, living a normal life, as we know it, is not an option.

Cocaine is a stimulant, which comes from the leaves of the coca plant. One of the most highly addictive forms of cocaine is crack. Simply stated, crack is a chemically altered form of cocaine that can be smoked. It takes only seconds for cocaine to enter the brain and for about six minutes a person may experience a rush of euphoria and a feeling of power and self-confidence.

It has been said that cocaine was once described like this: the second you do it, you want more. Cocaine addiction is as unique as its onset. People who use cocaine go through stages of social abuse and enter into the realm of addiction quicker than with any other drug, including such drugs as heroin, alcohol, PCP, or any combination of these. Cocaine causes debilitating effects both mentally and physically. Although some of the same symptoms occur with other drugs, the effects may not be seen for months, even years.

NEUROTRANSMISSION

To understand how drugs produce their effects, there must first be an understanding of how nerve cells interact with the molecules in certain drugs. The neuron, or nerve cell, is the basic building block of the nervous system. The neural system contains approximately 20 billion neurons, with 14 billion in the brain. Each neuron contains three important parts: (1) cell body, (2) dendrites, and (3) axon.

One of the reasons that drugs can exert such powerful control over a person's behavior is that they act directly on the brain and can override the cerebral cortex in controlling behavior. The feeling of pleasure is so important that there is a circuit of specialized nerve cells devoted to producing and regulating it. This neurotransmitter is called dopamine. The reason that pleasure, which is also called "reward," is such a powerful biological force for survival is that pleasure reinforces any behavior that elicits it. The activation of the pleasure circuit is an automatic and unconscious brain function. Life sustaining activities, such as eating and sex, activate this pleasure circuit called dopamine. Certain substances, such as alcohol, potently activate dopamine. This is the key reason why people repeatedly abuse drugs; drugs activate the pleasure circuit and triggers the brain to behave as if the substance is important for survival (Pohorecky, 1981).

NEUROTRANSMITTERS

There are many possible neurotransmitters; however, there are only a few that are affected by drugs: (1) acetylcholine, (2) catecholamines, (3) serotonin, (4) gamma-aminobutyric acid (GABA), (5) endorphins, and (6) glutamate. They fall into three categories: (1) excitatory neurotransmitters, which activate the postsynaptic cell, (2) inhibitory neurotransmitters, which depress the activity of the postsynaptic cell, and (3) neuromodulators, which modify the postsynaptic cell's response to other neurotransmitters. Neurons that release these substances form the basis of neural circuits that link different areas of the brain in a complex network of pathways and feedback loops.

Acetylcholine

Acetylcholine is the main neurotransmitter of a part of the autonomic nervous system called the parasympathetic system. Stimulation of the parasympathetic nervous system causes salivation, pupil contraction, slowing of the heart, speeding of the intestine, and other effects. It is synthesized by motor neurons almost exclusively, since few other cells can produce acetylcholine. Also, it is stored in synaptic vesicles where it waits to be released. A nerve impulse brings a depolarization of the plasma membrane of the nerve cell transmitting the message. This increases conductance for calcium ions. The inflow of calcium ions causes the synaptic vesicle to release acetylcholine into the synaptic cleft.

Acetyl receptor proteins located on the receiver cell(s) attach the acetylcholine. An ionic current causes the rapid depolarization that result in the message being transmitted. After acetylcholine is released, it is destroyed by the enzyme acetyl cholinesterase. Acetylcholine is produced at many sites, including the nucleus basalis of Meynert, a region located in basal forebrain. Its deficiency in the basal forebrain has been linked to memory disturbances in alcoholic

Korsakoff's syndrome (Arendt, 1993). Korsakoff patients have reduced cerebralspinal fluid levels of catecholamine metabolites that correlate with memory loss.

Dopamine

Dopamine is one of a number of neurotransmitters found in the CNS. It has received special attention from psychopharmacologists because of its apparent role in the regulation of mood and because of its role in the motivation and reward process. Although there are several dopamine systems in the brain, the mesolimbic dopamine system appears to be the most important for motivational processes.

Addictive drugs produce their potent effects on behavior by enhancing mesolimbic dopamine activity. Cells in the mesolimbic dopamine system are spontaneously active—this means that action potentials are constantly generated at a slow rate and small amounts of dopamine are released into the synaptic cleft. The levels of dopamine produced when the cells are active at this low rate may be responsible for maintaining normal affective tone and mood. This is why scientists speculate that some forms of clinical depression may be the result of unusually low dopamine levels.

Cocaine inhibits the reuptake of dopamine. This increases the availability of dopamine in the synapse and increases dopamine's action on the postsynaptic neurons. The enhanced dopamine activity produces mood elevation and euphoria. Cocaine's effect is usually quite short, prompting the user to repeatedly administer cocaine to reexperience its intense subjective effects.

Repeated use of psychomotor stimulants like cocaine produces change in the mesolimbic dopamine system. Specifically, repeated use of cocaine can deplete dopamine from this system, thereby causing normal rewards to lose their motivational significance.

PET studies show that cocaine works in large part by blocking dopamine transporter sites, which prevents reuptake of dopamine by the brain cells that release it. This allows higher concentrations of dopamine to remain available in the brain longer than normal. This abnormally long presence of dopamine in the brain is believed to cause the effects associated with cocaine use.

Other researchers have found that the cocaine abuser shows reduced dopamine responses to the drug in the striatum, a region of the brain linked to motivational control and reward. They also found abnormal increases in the level of dopamine response in the thalamus, a region of the brain that communicates sensory information (Wise, 1984).

Serotonin

Serotonin is a neurotransmitter released by signal-emitting neurons to subtly alter the function of signal-receiving neurons in a process called neuromodulation. Serotonin is produced in and released from neurons that originate within discrete regions or nuclei in the brain.

Many of the neurons are located at the base of the brain in two areas known as the raphe nucleus and the amygdala. The raphe nucleus influences brain functions related to attention, emotion, and motivation. The amygdala plays an important role in the control of emotions. In these brain areas, the axon endings of the serotonergic neurons secrete serotonin when activated.

Serotonin can influence mood states, thinking patterns, and even behaviors such as alcohol consumption. Its action at the synapses are tightly regulated by proteins called serotonin transporters, which remove the neurotransmitter from the synaptic cleft after a short period of time by transporting it back into the signal-emitting cell.

Serotonin can only affect neighboring neurons for a short period of time. Any interference with serotonin transporter function extends or diminishes the cell's exposure to serotonin, thereby disrupting the exquisite timing of nerve signals within the brain. The net result of such disruptions is abnormal brain activity, which can lead to psychological problems or mental illness. Inappropriate serotonin use in the brain has been linked to depression.

Animal studies have found acute alcohol exposure elevates serotonin levels within the brain, suggesting either that more serotonin is released from axons or that the neurotransmitter is cleared more slowly from the synapses (LeMarquand, Phil, and Benkelfat, 1994). This is said to contribute to alcohol's addicting effect.

Gamma-Aminobutyric Acid (GABA)

GABA is the main inhibitory neurotransmitter in the brain. GABA's high concentration in the hypothalamus suggests that it plays a significant role in hypothalamic–pituitary function. The hypothalamus is a region in the posterior section of the brain and is the regulating center for (instinctive) visceral functions such as sleep cycles, body temperature, and the activity of the pituitary gland, which is the master endocrine gland affecting all hormonal functions of the body.

GABA leads to a state of sedation and decreased anxiety. Some reports suggest that short-term alcohol exposure increases the inhibitory effect of GABA. Short-term alcohol consumption depresses brain functioning by altering the balance between inhibitory and excitatory neurotransmission. Alcohol can act as a depressant by increasing inhibitory neurotransmission, decreasing excitatory neurotransmission, or through a combination of both.

Alcohol's depressant effect on neurons may be associated with some of the behavioral manifestations of intoxication. Alcohol consumption is initially accompanied by decreased attention, alterations in memory, mood changes, and drowsiness. According to Deitrich and Erwin (1996), continued acute consumption may result in lethargy, confusion, amnesia, loss of sensation, difficulty in breathing, and death. Alcohol's excitatory action (e.g., reduction of social inhibitions) appears to be caused, at least in part, by suppression of inhibitory neurotransmitter systems (Pohorecky, 1981).

Endorphins

Chemical painkillers known as endorphins and enkephalins are produced naturally in the body. They are polypeptides, able to bind to the neuroreceptors in the brain to give pain relief. This effect appears to be responsible for the so-called runner's high, and the temporary loss of pain when severe injury occurs.

Four groups of endorphins, alpha, beta, gamma, and sigma, have been identified. Alpha-endorphin contains sixteen amino acids, Beta-endorphin contains thirty-one amino acids, Gamma-endorphin contains seventeen amino acids, and Sigma-endorphin contains twenty-seven amino acids. Polypeptides with greater than fifty amino acids in their chains are called proteins.

The enkephalins are found in the thalamus of the brain and in parts of the spinal cord that transmit pain impulses. The amino acid sequence of enkephalin is found in the longer amino acid sequence of the endorphin.

A chemical called substance P, a polypeptide with eleven amino acids, has been found to transmit pain impulses to the brain. Endorphins may act to prevent the release of substance P, which may account for the sedating of endogenous endorphins and narcotics given exogenously, such as cocaine and morphine (Deitrich and Erwin, 1996).

Glutamate

Glutamate is an amino acid. Molecules of this type are the building blocks of proteins. Because all cells in the body, including neurons, produce proteins, glutamate is present throughout the brain in relatively high concentrations.

Glutamatergic neurotransmission plays a pivotal role in brain function throughout the lifespan. Glutamate relays excitatory signals between neurons that form specific circuits and whose activation leads to sensations, thoughts, and actions.

Glutamatergic neurotransmission also occurs in the synaptic connections that mediate the brain's response to various environmental and developmental influences. Throughout life, some forms of learning and memory, as well as higher cognitive functions likely depend on normal glutamatergic activity. In addition, the brain's compensatory responses to certain injuries are probably mediated by glutamate-dependent signaling (Parker and Noble, 1977).

To prevent overstimulation of neurons, excitatory neurotransmission is tightly regulated. The loss of these regulatory influences may result in pathological conditions, such as seizures or neurodegenerative disease. Alcohol consumption inhibits glutamatergic neurotransmission and may cause chronic alcohol consumption, cognitive dysfunction, physical dependence—which may lead to FAS.

PRENATAL CONSIDERATIONS

Marijuana

There have been reports of an association between prenatal marijuana exposure and smaller size at birth; however, these reports have been offset by reports that have found no such effect. The effects of marijuana exposure on the brain have been found in older children. Three-year-old children showed significant effects of first- and second-trimester exposure to marijuana on the composite score of the Stanford-Binet Intelligence Scale, as well as on those portions of the scale that measures short-term memory, verbal reasoning, and abstract/visual reasoning (Day et al., 1991). These children also showed the same results at age six. Overall, the results suggest that prenatal exposure to marijuana has significant effects on sleep and, at older ages, on measures of intellectual development and behavior (Day et al., 1991). There are few or no effects of prenatal exposure on growth or physical development.

Cocaine

Prenatal cocaine exposure has been associated with decreased length of gestation and increased rate of prematurity. Researchers have also reported decreased weight, length, and head circumference in cocaine-exposed newborns. Withdrawal symptoms in newborns may include jitteriness, poor muscle tone, and poor feeding. Infants are reported to (1) be fussy and inconsolable, (2) lose a state of control when stimulated with touch or voice, and (3) look away when their gaze is engaged (Chasnoff et al., 1992). Investigators have demonstrated significant effects of cocaine use during pregnancy; however, there are few studies on the long-term effect of cocaine exposure.

Alcohol

FAS is the leading known cause of mental retardation. According to Day (1995), studies of population groups in the United States have most consistently found rates ranging from 1 to 3 per 1,000 live births.

The criteria for diagnosis of FAS require at least one feature from each of the following three categories:

1. Prenatal and postnatal growth retardation, with abnormally small-for-age weight, length, and/or head circumference.
2. CNS disorders, with signs of abnormal brain functioning, delays in behavioral development, and/or intellectual impairment.
3. At least two features from the following: abnormal craniofacial features—small head, small eyes, or short eye openings, or a poorly developed philtrum (the groove above the upper lip), thin upper lip, short nose, or flattened mid-facial area.

Other abnormalities have been reported with FAS, including the following: crossed eyes (strabismus) and nearsightedness, malformations of the ears, heart murmurs, liver and kidney problems, retarded bone growth and skeletal defects, increases in upper respiratory infections and middle ear infections, and undescended testicles and hernias. Prenatally alcohol-exposed with birth defects that do not meet all three criteria for a FAS diagnosis may be categorized as having suspected "fetal alcohol effects." These adverse consequences of maternal alcohol use include growth retardation and are estimated to be about three times more frequent than FAS (Day, 1995). In absence of growth retardation or congenital abnormalities, children born to women who drank excessively during pregnancy appear to be at increased risk for attention deficit disorders with hyperactivity, fine-motor impairment and clumsiness, as well as subtle delays in motor performance and speech disorders.

Can the Brain Recover from the Effects of Drugs?

According to Jernigan et al. (1991), prolonged alcohol abuse is associated with brain damage and corresponding changes in mental functioning. Brain-imaging techniques such as MRI and CT scans have provided evidence that alcoholism causes brain changes. One of the most serious neurological outcomes of alcoholism is Kosakoff's syndrome, which is characterized by memory deficits, such as anterograde amnesia, which is an inability to remember new information for more than a few seconds, as well as other cognitive impairments. Despite these deficits, the patient's intellectual abilities (as measured by IQ tests) remain relatively intact because much of the information and ability assesses by an IQ test is acquired in the distant past and because patients with Korsakoff's syndrome usually retain memories formed before the onset of prolonged heavy drinking. Other procedures such as the PET scan and event-related potentials (ERPs), which measure the electrical activity of groups of nerve cells in various parts of the brain, show evidence of abnormal brain functioning and brain shrinkage. Regions vulnerable to damage, with resulting impairment in mental functioning include the cerebellum, limbic system, diencephalons, and regions of the cerebral cortex. This is of great concern because innumerable neuronal pathways interconnect these and other areas of the brain and damage to one structure or system may affect another structure or system.

Finally, Hyman (1998) states, "Prolonged drug use can change the brain in fundamental and possibly permanent ways. Some changes that can happen in the brain may be irreversible, especially (some) emotional memories." Oscar-Berman (1992) completed a study designed to test the emotional functioning of patients with Korsakoff's syndrome. Researchers used photographs of facial expressions conveying four emotions: happiness, sadness, anger, and neutrality, along with recordings of sentences having intonations or semantic meanings conveying the same four emotions. The results indicate significant deficits in visual and auditory emotional perception and memory. Hyman (1998) states, "that just as people with strokes are able to, addicts can recover by using parts of their brain that were not affected by drugs."

REFERENCES

Arendt, T. (1993). The Cholinergic Deafferenation of Cerebral Cortex Induced by Chronic Consumption of Alcohol: Reversal by Cholinergic Drugs and Transplantation.

Bernstein, D. and E. Tiegerman (1989). *Language and Communication Disorders in Children.* New York: Macmillan Publishing Company.

Chasnoff, I., Griffith, D., Freier, C., and J. Murray (1992). Cocaine/Polydrug Use in Pregnancy: Two-Year Follow-Up. *Pediatrics.* 89, 284-289.

Day, N. (1995). Editorail: Research on the Effects of Prenatal Alcohol Exposure—a New Direction. *American Journal of Public Health.* 85, 1614-1615.

Day, N., Sambamoorthi, U., Taylor, P., Richardson, G., Robles, N., Scher, M., Stoffer, D., Cornelius, M., and D. Jasperse (1991). Prenatal Marijuana Use and Neonatal Outcome. *Neurotoxicology and Terotology.* 13, 329-334.

Deitrich, R. and V. Erwin (1996). *Pharmacological Effects of Ethanol on the Nervous System.* Boca Raton: CRC Press.

Hyman, S. Can the Addicted Brain Change Back. Brookhaven National Laboratory Center of Imaging and Neurosciences. Wysivg://96http://www.pbs.org/wnet/closethome/science/html/change.html (October 25, 1998).

Jernigan, T., Schafer, K., Butlers, N., and L. Cermak (1991). Magnetic Resonance Imaging of Alcoholic Korsakoff Patients. *Neuropsychopharmacology.* 4, 175-186.

LeMarquand, D., Phil, R., and C. Benkelfat (1994). Serotonin and Alcohol Intake, Abuse, Dependence. *Biological Psychiatry.* 36, 326-337.

Oscar-Breman, M. (1992). Alcoholism and Asymmetries of Brain Function. *Alcohol Health Research World.* 16, 273-279.

Parker, E.S. and E.P. Noble (1977). Alcohol Consumption and Cognitive Functioning in Social Drinkers. *Journal of Studies on Alcohol.* 38 (7), 1224-1232.

Pohorecky, L. (1981). The Interaction of Alcohol and Stress: A Review. *Neuroscience Behavior Review.* 5, 209-229.

Porjesz, B. and H. Begleiter (1981). Human Evoked Brain Potentials and Alcohol. *Alcoholism: Clinical and Experimental Research.* 5 (2), 304-317.

Ron, M.A. (1979). Organic Psychosyndromes in Chronic Alcoholics. *British Journal of Addiction.* 74, 353-358.

Tarter, R.E. and K.L. Edwards (1986). Multifactorial Etiology of Neuropsychological Impairment in Alcoholics. *Alcoholism: Clinical and Experimental Research.* 10 (2), 128-135.

U.S. Department of Health and Human Services. Marijuana: Fact Parents Need to Know. (1995). National Institute on Drug Abuse. Washington, DC: U.S. Government Printing Office.

Wilkinson, D.A. (1987). CT Scan and Neuropsychological Assessments of Alcoholism. In: Parsons, O.A., Butters, N., and P.E. Nathan, eds. *Neuropsychology of Alcoholism: Implications for Diagnosis and Treatment.* New York: The Guilford Press. 78-102.

Wise, R. (1984). Neural Mechanisms of the Reinforcing Action of Cocaine. National Institute on Drug Abuse. Washington, DC: U.S. Government Printing Office.

Chapter 4

HIV and Communication Disorders

PEDIATRIC POPULATIONS

As people with HIV and AIDS live longer, communication disorders that occur as a direct or indirect consequence of HIV infection are more commonplace. Speech, language, and hearing problems frequently result as the virus attacks the CNS, with nearly 100 percent of its manifestations on the head and neck. These problems—some of which were initially attributed to apathy, forgetfulness, and depression—are now recognized as serious communication disorders that can affect all aspects of a person's life. An ever-increasing group infected by HIV-1 is the pediatric population. Data presented by Scott and Layton (1997) revealed that 4,710 cases of AIDS in children under 13 years of age had been reported in the United States, and that HIV ranks among the 10 leading causes of death of children ages 1 to 4 years. Furthermore, racial distributions show that, in both the adult and pediatric populations, the prevalence of infected American minorities far exceeds that of infected European Americans (Scott and Layton, 1997). It is more important to note that available person, place, and time distributions suggest that most children with HIV are African American.

Children acquire HIV in the following four ways: parenterally by shared contaminated needles or sharp objects, accidental blood exposure, blood transfusions, and tissue or organ transplantation; sexually by infected semen, genital secretions, or blood; or through breastfeeding. However, it is transmission during the perinatal period, that

HIV, Substance Abuse, and Communication Disorders in Children
© 2007 by The Haworth Press, Inc. All rights reserved.
doi:10.1300/5438_04

is, transmission transplacentally from mother to fetus, or at delivery by contact with infected blood or vaginal secretions, that is the primary way children become infected with HIV.

Given the nature of HIV transmission from infected mothers to their children, one might assume that all children born to HIV-positive women acquire the virus. However, approximately 60 to 75 percent of these children (referred to as "HIV-exposed") lose their maternally acquired antibodies and serovert, or change their HIV antibody status from positive to negative (Scott and Layton, 1997). Also important is the fact that the birth incidence of mother-to-child transmission of HIV is reduced from 25-40 percent to 8 percent when the mother received AZT during pregnancy (Scott and Layton, 1997).

In children, AIDS most frequently causes neurologic sequellae. Neurologic sequallae may be the result of direct invasion of the more mature brain of parenterally infected populations (thereby causing HIV encephalopathy, for example). Damage may also be the result of HIV's direct invasion of the developing brains or the nervous systems of perinatally infected child population, yielding possible atrophy or microencephaly. Furthermore, neuropathologies may include opportunistic infections of the CNS, such as cytomegalovirus (CMV) and cryptococcus (Scott and Layton, 1997).

Since HIV infection affects the brain, spinal cord, and nerves, the resulting cognitive and motor changes can affect communication. Some language disorders that can result from HIV infection in adults are aphasia (the loss or impairment of the power to use or comprehend words, usually resulting from a brain lesion), confabulations (filling in gaps of memory by free fabrication), and language confusion (usually refers to a delay in the development of language in children when understanding and/or use of grammatical constructions and vocabulary is delayed) (ASHA, 1997). Language disorders that are unique to pediatric HIV patients include elective mutism (ongoing inability to produce speech in specific situations, usually connected with hysteria, inordinate inhibition, or other emotional, rather than physiological, factors), and pragmatic language disorder or delay (a disorder related to or a delay in the development of the skills necessary for appropriate use of language with various social contexts, including the "rules" of conversation and adaptation of tone and word choice based on the purpose) (ASHA, 1997).

In addition to neuropathologies with language dysfunction as an outcome, oral pathologies are common among pediatric HIV-infected populations. Typical oral manifestations consist of salivary gland disease and parotid enlargement found in as many as 30 percent of the infected children (ASHA, 1997). Research indicates that otitis media is prevalent in the pediatric HIV-infected population (Scott and Layton, 1997). It is well known that there is a high correlation with chronic otitis media and language development delay.

In a study by Coplan et al. (1998), a comparison of language development in infected and in exposed but uninfected infants in young children was conducted. Global language scores were significantly lower for subjects with HIV infection, compared with uninfected subjects (89.3 vs. 96.2, on the Mann-Whitney U test) (Coplan et al., 1998). Seven of the nine subjects with HIV infection manifested deterioration of language function. Three subjects with HIV infection and language deterioration showed improvement in language almost immediately after the initiation of antiretroviral drug treatment (Coplan et al., 1998). Magnetic resonance imaging or computed tomography of the brain were performed in six of seven infected subjects with language deterioration, and findings were normal in all six (Coplan et al., 1998). Thus, Coplan et al. (1998) concluded that language deterioration occurs commonly in infants and young children with HIV infection, and is seen frequently in the absence of abnormalities on neurologic examination or CNS imaging, and may precede evidence of deterioration in global cognitive ability. Coplan et al. (1998) also concluded that periodic assessment of language development should be added to the developmental monitoring of infants and young children with HIV infection as a means of monitoring disease progression and the efficacy of drug treatment.

In a study by Wolters et al. (1997), it was determined that expressive language was consistently more impaired than receptive language over a twenty-four-month longitudinal assessment. This supported an earlier finding that HIV differentially affected expressive language in children with symptomatic disease (Wolters et al., 1997). In contrast to Coplan et al. (1998), the subjects in the study conducted by Wolters et al. (1997) declined significantly in receptive and expressive language after twenty-four months despite antiretroviral therapy, although overall cognitive function remained stable. Thus, it was concluded by Wolters et al. (1997) that functioning in some domains may be more vulnerable to the effects of HIV, and global measures of cognitive ability may mask such differential changes in specific brain functions.

In a study by Tardieu et al. (1995), thirty-three children who had been vertically infected with HIV-1 and had reached the age of six years were studied and tested for school achievement. Of these thirty-three children, twenty-four were also tested for cognitive abilities, fine motor skills, and emotional adaptation (Tardieu et al., 1995). Children with normal school achievement had a higher percentage of circulating CD4+ lymphocytes during the course of infection (Tardieu et al., 1995). Thus, it was concluded that children whose HIV-1 infection is maternally acquired have better cognitive abilities and school achievement than was initially thought, and that the percentage of circulating CD+ lymphocytes during the first year of life appears to be predictive of future school adaptation or cognitive abilities (Tardieu et al., 1995).

All children with HIV do not experience the same communication disorder, just as they do not acquire the same opportunistic infections or clinical manifestations of HIV/AIDS. It is important to note, however, that the mode of HIV transmission, and, therefore, age at infection, appears to affect the subsequent outcomes presenting in immunocompromised child populations. It has been reported that hemophiliac children who acquire HIV infection, secondary to transfusion, differ from infants with perinatally acquired HIV (Scott and Layton, 1997). The hemophiliac HIV-infected child population has a premorbid history of language similar to nonhemophiliac populations, whereas infants infected from birth, or within the first two years, typically lack this period of normalcy (Scott and Layton, 1997).

Scott and Layton (1997) noted in their study that measuring risk for communication disorders can be a risky business for three important reasons: (1) communication disorders are often secondary or tertiary to other conditions and actually may be symptoms of primary conditions, (2) a communication disorder may be one of multiple outcomes from known risk factors, and (3) the clinical continuum of mild to severe communication changes over time along this continuum may make case ascertainment difficult.

These principles are applicable to HIV. First, HIV-related neuro-pathologies, opportunistic infections, and other clinical manifestations may be viewed as primary conditions experienced by children with HIV. Infected children exhibit more voice disorders, dysphagia, and language dysfunction, which, therefore, may be considered secondary or tertiary conditions and/or symptoms of primary conditions (Scott and Layton, 1997). Second, communication disorders demonstrated by children with and/or exposed to HIV may, in part, be a result of known risk factors for HIV transmission; other risk factors confound the attempt to measure the effect of HIV on communication (Scott and Layton, 1997). For example, the high proportion of women who acquire HIV via intravenous drug use frequently give birth a population of children who are exposed to polysubstances, in addition to HIV in utero. This then makes it difficult to determine whether the outcome of the communication disorder is caused by exposure to any or all of the polysubstances, the HIV virus alone, or perhaps a combination of the two.

Third, HIV is a progressive disease. Children with the infection change over time in terms of severity of immunosuppression. Therefore, changes in the speech production and communication disorders may be exhibited as the disease progresses (Scott and Layton, 1997). Thus, it is reasonable to state that modes of transmission and age of onset may affect the variety of presenting opportunistic infections and clinical manifestations, which in turn may affect developmental outcomes.

Another relevant factor that needs to be addressed is that the environments of HIV-infected children can be unstable, for the children may be shuffled between biological parents, guardians, or foster families (Scott and Layton, 1997). The children's environments may also be affected by the age of the caregivers and by the number of siblings at home. Living with HIV means coping with the stresses that can accompany the infection, including painful medical treatments, frequent hospitalizations, and disruptions in routing. Stress can come from parents who, themselves, are at increased risk for chronic illness and/or substance dependence. If so, they may be incapable of providing adequate or consistent child care. Finally, families and infected children must continuously face the social stigma associated with HIV. Unfortunately, all of these stresses that may occur simultaneously in the lives of children with HIV may be associated with speech and language development and, therefore, may affect the severity of speech and language disorders (Scott and Layton, 1997).

In conclusion, professionals need to broaden their examinations from individual puzzle pieces to the expanded epidemiologic view of how the pieces combine to complete the whole puzzle. Epidemiologic principles require researchers to analyze the individual pieces as they relate to the whole. These interrelationships are complex and can broaden the perspective of those professionals concerned with the way speech, language, swallowing, voice, and otologic disorders fit within the overall puzzle of the immunocompromised populations that have been recognized only recently. To understand the full implications of HIV-1 on language disorders, one has to look at the child's complete situation before making diagnostic judgments.

REFERENCES

ASHA (1997). Communication Disorders and HIV: The HIV Treatment Community's Guide to Working with Audiologists and Speech-Language Pathologists. Available at: www.iapac.org/clinmgt/commdis/ashabrochure.html.

Coplan, J., Contello, K.A., Cunningham, C.K., Weiner, L.B., Dye, T.D., Roberge, L., Wojtowycz, M.A., and K. Kirkwood (1998). Early Language Development in Children Exposed to or Infected with Human Immunodeficiency Virus. *Pediatrics.* 102(1), e8.

Scott, G.S. and T.L. Layton (1997). Epidemiologic Principles in Studies of Infectious Disease Outcomes: Pediatric HIV as a Model. *Journal of Communication Disorders.* 30(4), 303-322.

Tardieu, M., Mayaux, M.J., Seibel, N., Funck-Brentano, I., Straub, E., Teglas, J.P., and S. Blanche (1995). Cognitive Assessment of School-Age Children Infected with Maternally Transmitted Human Immunodeficiency Virus Type 1. *Journal of Pediatrics.* 126(3), 375-379.

Wolters, P.L., Brouwers, P., Civitello, L., and H.A. Moss (1997). Receptive and Expressive Language Function of Children with Symptomatic HIV Infection and Relationship with Disease Parameters: A Longitudinal 24-Month Follow-up Study. *AIDS.* 11(9), 1135-1144.

Chapter 5

The Impact of HIV Exposure
on Linguistic Functioning in Children

Lemmietta G. McNeilly

INTRODUCTION

Children born exposed to HIV present with several at-risk characteristics that cause them to be at risk for delays in language development. This chapter provides an overview of prenatal HIV exposure and the characteristics of the groups of children with exposure. In addition, descriptive linguistic features as analyzed by the author are discussed. Considerations for speech-language pathologists regarding intervention and prevention of delays are also addressed.

BACKGROUND OF HIV IN CHILDREN

The number of HIV-positive children identified in the United States is decreasing daily (CDC, 1999). This phenomenon is attributable to the successful prescribing of antiretroviral treatment to mothers during pregnancy and delivery concluding with the baby's receipt of ARV treatment for the first six weeks of life. Speech-language pathologists who provide evaluative and management services to this population have done so without much clinical information available in the literature regarding specific communication delays and disorders typically identified in individuals with HIV infection.

HIV, Substance Abuse, and Communication Disorders in Children
© 2007 by The Haworth Press, Inc. All rights reserved.
doi:10.1300/5438_05

In 1997, the Public Health Service (PHS) reported that AIDS/HIV had become the fifth leading cause of death in children under five years of age. HIV infection continues to present a challenge to health care providers, including speech-language pathologists. The high frequency of neurodevelopmental problems associated with HIV infection in children poses special dilemmas to those who provide services to children with developmental disabilities (Cohen and Diamond, 1992). Since HIV infection is a progressive disease, early indicators of lost or plateaued skills may provide good diagnostic information for health management teams when no physiological or neurological factors are yet clearly evident (Meyers and Weitzman, 1991).

Many young children with HIV infection are living longer lives before they progress to AIDS and they exhibit speech and language delays and disorders. It is, therefore, important for specialists from many disciplines to know the specific characteristics of developmental delays that may be exhibited by members of this population. Cognitive, fine and gross motor, and speech and language skills are a few of the areas in which deficits have been reported in the majority of children with HIV infection (Pizzo and Wilfert, 1991). Service providers also need to collaborate and coordinate early intervention services offered to these children so that their developmental needs may be addressed and managed early and appropriately to reduce disabilities. More specific information is, therefore, needed to enhance the services available and accessible to these children.

TRANSMISSION

HIV can be transmitted from infected mothers to infants perinatally during pregnancy, delivery, or breastfeeding. A small percentage of children have been reported to acquire HIV via other routes, such as blood transfusion—2 percent, or sexual abuse—2 percent (Fleming, Gwinn, and Oxtoby, 1992). The subjects in this study will target children with perinatally transmitted HIV infection only.

The majority, 92 percent, of the African-American pediatric HIV cases reported to the CDC were born to mothers with or at risk for HIV infection. The primary way that perinatal transmission of HIV occurs is when the virus is transmitted in utero from the mother to the fetus (Lewis et al., 1990).

Speech-language pathologists who provide evaluative and management services to HIV-positive children have done so without much clinical information available in the literature regarding specific communication delays and disorders typically identified in young children with HIV infection. In addition, children living with biological families are impacted by the psychosocial and emotional elements of living with HIV. These factors may also affect language development. A significant number of children exposed to HIV do not live with their biological mothers and reside in either foster or adoptive homes.

CLASSIFICATION OF HIV INFECTION IN CHILDREN

The spectrum of HIV-related diseases led to the development of a pediatric classification system by the CDC (Exhibit 5.1). Previous terms, such as AIDS-related complex (ARC) and pre-AIDS, used to describe children considered to be less severely ill than full-blown AIDS have been replaced by a specific classification system developed by the CDC (1987). This system has undergone two revisions with the most recent occurring in 1994.

EXHIBIT 5.1.

1994 Revised Human Immunodeficiency Virus Pediatric
Classification System: Clinical Categories

Category N: Not Symptomatic

Children who have no signs or symptoms considered to be the result of HIV infection or who have only one of the conditions listed in category A.

Category A: Mildly Symptomatic

Children with two or more of the following conditions but none of the conditions listed in categories B and C:

(continued)

(continued)

- Lymphadenopathy
- Hepatomegaly
- Splenomegaly
- Dermatitis
- Parotitis
- Recurrent or persistent upper respiratory infection, sinusitis, or otitis media

Category B: Moderately Symptomatic

Children who have symptomatic conditions other than listed for category A or category C that are attributed to HIV infection. Examples of conditions in clinical category B include but are not limited to the following:

- Anemia, neutopenia, or thrombocytopenia persisting > 30 days
- Bacterial meningitis, pneumonia, or sepsis (single episode)
- Candidasis, oropharyngeal persisting for two months
- Cardiomyopathy
- Cytomegalovirus infection with onset before age 1 month
- Diarrhea, recurrent or chronic
- Hepatitis
- Herpes simplex virus (HSV) stomatitis, recurrent (i.e., more that two episodes within 1 year)
- HSV bronchitis, pneumonitis, or esophagitis with onset before age 1 month
- Herpes roster involving at least two distinct episodes or more than one dermatome
- Leiomyosarcoma
- Lymphoid interstitial pneumonia (LIP) or pulmonary lymphoid hyperplasia complex
- Nephropathy
- Nocardosis
- Fever lasting > 1 month
- Toxoplasmosis with onset before age 1 month
- Varicella, disseminated (i.e., complicated chicken pox)

Category C: Severely Symptomatic

Children who have any condition listed in the 1987 surveillance case definition for acquired immunodeficiency syndrome, with the exception of LIP (which is a category B condition) (CDC, 1994).

Source: Adapted from 1994 Revised Classification System for Human Immunodeficiency Virus Infection in Children Less Than 13 Years of Age. *MMWR,* 43 (RR-12) 1-10.

Children under the ages of thirteen who are infected with the human immunodeficiency virus are classified according to the Pediatric HIV Classification system developed by the CDC (Table 5.1). Children who are asymptomatic and test positive are classified as HIV P-1. Children born to mothers who are HIV positive and, therefore, tested positive for the HIV antibody, but who after losing their mother's antibodies, have seroreverted, are classified as P-3 (CDC, 1987). Seroreversion refers to the loss of a mother's antibodies and this occurs when the baby is between nine and eighteen months of age. The current Pediatric HIV classification is summarized in Table 5.1.

DEMOGRAPHICS OF POPULATION

HIV infection affects a significant number of minority ethnic groups. The percent of cumulative perinatally acquired pediatric AIDS cases reported through June 1999 by ethnicity included 61 percent African American, 23 percent Hispanic, and 14 percent white, and less than 1 percent either Asian or Native Americans. Gender distribution is essentially equal. Of the 1991 pediatric AIDS cases reported through June 1999, 92 percent are perinatally acquired (CDC, 1999).

The percent of pediatric HIV cases born to a mother with/at risk for HIV infection through June 1999 by ethnicity included 66 percent African American, 12 percent Hispanic, and 21 percent white, and less than 1 percent either Asian or Native Americans. It is projected that minorities will account for an increasing proportion of cases among women and children, in the coming years (CDC, 1999).

TABLE 5.1. Pediatric HIV Classification Summary

	Clinical Categories			
Immunologic Categories	N:No signs/ symptoms	A:Mild signs/ symptoms	B:Moderate signs/ symptoms	C:Severe signs/ symptoms
1. No evidence of suppression	N1	A1	B1	C1
2. Evidence of moderate suppression	N2	A2	B2	C2
3. Severe suppression	N3	A3	B3	C3

Source: Centers for Disease Control (1994).

NEUROLOGICAL PROFILE

Infants born to HIV-infected mothers are at increased risk for a variety of additional factors that can adversely affect development (Speigel and Mayers, 1991). Low birth weight (Vohr and Hack, 1982), poor prenatal care, and fetal alcohol and drug exposure (Clarren and Smith, 1978; Lifschitz, Wilson, and Smith, 1985; Rosen and Johnson, 1982) have been shown to correlate with significant neurodevelopmental delays. In none of these cases is a progressive deteriorating course described.

HIV encephalopathy is central to the pediatric neurological profile. The term, encephalopathy, is used in clinical settings to describe the changes in motor and mental status seen in children with documented systemic HIV infection. The encephalopathy is frequently manifested by one or a combination of features that may occur in either static or a progressive course, at varying rates of deterioration. Some of these features include loss of previously acquired milestones or failure to attain them at the expected age, intellectual deficits, impaired brain growth, and seizures and extrapyramidal tract signs (Cohen and Diamond, 1992).

High epidemiological incidence figures for HIV seropositivity and consequent infection among newborns as well as very high prevalence figure of 90 percent neurodevelopmental impairment (motor and cognitive deficits combined) were found in separate studies conducted with the same inner city population (Cogo et al., 1990; Tardieu et al., 1989, 1987).

DEVELOPMENTAL DELAYS

Developmental delays are the predominant sequelae of HIV infection in children and are most apparent in the areas of motor and language skills acquisition (Spiegel and Mayers, 1991). Children with prenatally acquired HIV infection are additionally at risk to the acquisition of other factors that adversely affect development, including prenatal drug exposure. Nearly all children with HIV infection need rehabilitative services, particularly in the areas of phonology, language, and social interaction. The literature has indicated gross speech and language delays in the symptomatic HIV-infected pediatric population.

The predominant feature of AIDS in children is a pattern of developmental delay in infancy and progressive cognitive impairments in older children. Developmental delays are present in the majority of symptomatic children with HIV infection, with reports of involvement ranging from 60 to 90 percent of children (Belman et al., 1998; Falloon et al., 1989; Ultmann et al., 1985). However, asymptomatic HIV-positive children are typically not identified early because they are not routinely tested for presence of the virus.

The extent of the developmental and cognitive impairment in children appears directly related to the site and extent of HIV infection in the CNS (Falloon et al., 1989). Acquired microcephaly, radiological evidence of cerebral atrophy, and other indicators of direct brain involvement have been widely reported (Falloon et al., 1989; and Ultmann et al., 1985). Specific deficits have also been described in the areas of perceptual and visual motor skills, receptive and expressive language skills (McCardle et al., 1991; Ultmann et al., 1985), as well as prelinguistic skills in younger children (Nozyce et al., 1989).

SPEECH AND LANGUAGE CONCERNS

A few studies have documented communication delays identified in children with HIV infection. The frequent finding of hearing loss (Hopkins, 1989) and deficits in language development are common. The literature includes documentation of several types of oral communication difficulties. These include oral motor difficulties characterized by phonological errors, raspy and strained vocal quality exacerbated with candidasis in the oral-laryngeal cavity, expressive language delays, and receptive language delays—sporadically as well as expressive—receptive language discrepancies (Seidel, 1992; McCardle et al., 1991; Watchel et al., 1989; Hittleman et al., 1991; Levenson et al., 1991; Pressman, 1992; Wolters et al., 1989; Wolters et al., 1994; McKinney and Robertson, 1993; Wolters, 1992; Wolters et al., 1995, 1997). Clinicians must be aware of the environmental and cultural context of pediatric AIDS as well as the clinical profiles.

Language skills are central to the development of social functioning in childhood, and the loss of developmental milestones often indicates progression of HIV disease in the absence of other clinical signs. Therefore, early identification and subsequent early intervention are particularly important to children with HIV infection (Spiegel and Mayers, 1991).

Descriptions in the literature of specific language skills in children who are HIV exposed between the ages of fifteen and thirty-six months are severely limited. Thus, more research is needed to label and describe the parameters of phonological, expressive, and receptive language features exhibited in children with HIV infection. Pediatric AIDS strikes a population already devastated by multiple psychosocial stresses (Spiegel and Mayers, 1991).

McNeilly conducted a study in 1998 to provide a descriptive analysis of the phonological, receptive, and expressive language skills displayed by children ages eighteen to thirty-six months of age with HIV infection. The results of the McNeilly study increased the knowledge base regarding communication profiles of children with perinatal exposure to HIV. The results of the study provide speech– language pathologists with some descriptive information regarding receptive and expressive language skills of young children with perinatal HIV exposure. In addition, living environments were analyzed to determine any significant correlations (McNeilly, 1998).

McNeilly's study investigated the receptive and expressive language skills displayed by three groups of subjects, ages fifteen to thirty-six months of age born to mothers with HIV infection. Information was obtained regarding the impact of perinatal HIV exposure and prenatal antiretroviral treatment on receptive and expressive language skills in this age group as measured by the Preschool Language Scale-3 (PLS-3). In addition, the interaction of HIV classification and absence or presence of prenatal antiretroviral treatment on expressive, receptive, and overall language skills were analyzed.

The results indicate a number of significant findings, which were summarized, based upon HIV classification, prenatal antiretroviral treatment, and biological mother living in the home and MLU (McNeilly, 1998).

HIV CLINICAL CLASSIFICATION RESULTS

1. All groups of subjects achieved scores that fell below the mean on the three subscales of the PLS-3: auditory comprehension, expressive communication, and total language.
2. The PLS-3 scores on the auditory comprehension, expressive communication, and total language subscales exhibited by subjects in HIV class A (mild) were higher than the scores exhibited by subjects in the E (exposed) and B (moderate) classes.
3. Subjects with prenatal exposure that seroreverted to HIV-negative status exhibited language skills that were below HIV-positive subjects in group A with mild symptomology.

Prenatal Antiretroviral Treatment Results

1. Prenatal Antiretroviral treatment was not significant for subjects as measured by results of the PLS-3 Auditory Comprehension Expressive Communication and Total Language subscales.

Mother Living in the Home Results

1. When adjusted for age, mother living in the home is statistically significant for results of the auditory comprehension standard scores and age equivalent scores and total language age equivalent scores on the PLS-3.
2. Mother living in the home is not significant for MLU.

MLU Results

1. MLU is significant for age.
2. MLU is significant for HIV exposure when adjusted for age.
3. MLU is not significant for ARV or mother living in home.
4. The interaction between HIV class and prenatal ARV treatment is not statistically significant for the linguistic variable MLU.

TREATMENT OF LANGUAGE DISORDERS

Documented delays in the expressive and receptive aspects of linguistic functioning for children with HIV infection are present in the literature (McCardle et al., 1991; Wolters et al., 1997; McNeilly, 1998). Delays in expressive language skills are reported more often than are receptive delays (McCardle et al., 1991; Wolters et al., 1997; McNeilly, 1998). Functional usage of language is also reported as an area that warrants intervention in a significant number of children living with HIV infection.

Expressive language delays exhibited by children with HIV have been characterized by reduced/limited vocabulary, simple sentence structure, immature morphological features, and higher single word responses than expected for chronological age (McNeilly, 1998). Receptive language delays are visible in children's comprehension of complex syntactical utterances, that is, difficulty in processing long or multiple part messages.

Many children from culturally and linguistically different backgrounds who are referred for language assessment do not have disorders. However, some children from culturally/linguistically different backgrounds do exhibit language disorders. For these children, it is the speech-language pathologist's responsibility to provide intervention in a culturally appropriate manner (McNeilly and Coleman, 2000).

There are several morphological, syntactical, and pragmatic components of English present in America. The dialectal variations and vernacular usage of English spoken in different regions of the country and by members of various ethnically diverse populations need to be validated based upon the community in which the child resides. An examiner who is not familiar with the specific features of the dialects spoken might misinterpret communication behaviors as disorders when they are dialectal or cultural differences (McNeilly and Coleman, 2000). These issues are also relevant for children by HIV infection.

Language treatment strategies may involve a variety of approaches dependent upon the age and level of function for the child. Whole language is a popular approach to intervention that targets functional usage of vocabulary within naturalistic contexts, resulting in repetitive functional opportunities to teach and learn new vocabulary both receptively and expressively.

REHABILITATION CONSIDERATIONS

Binder and Castagnino (1993) cited rehabilitation needs of HIV-infected infants and children, management of rehabilitation needs, and support for families and caretakers. Rehabilitation needs of children should be based on the child's age and presenting symptomotology. Infants and children without neurologic deficits may have other hospitalizations. Children with progressive neurologic deficits due to encephalopathy or other neurologic problems may need therapy to reduce or hinder further deterioration of function. Infants and children with static neurologic and developmental deficits and complications of premature birth, intrauterine drug, or alcohol exposure, metabolic or endocrine problems, or environmental deprivation tend to demonstrate mild spasticity, failure to thrive, and significant cognitive impairments.

Clinical management of the developmental needs of HIV-positive infants and children is best addressed by a team whose members provide services in a clinic setting, school system, or community based setting (Cohen and Diamond, 1992; Crocker, 1989). Most children need physical therapy, and practically all infants need occupational therapy and speech-language therapy because of global developmental delays and feeding problems. Because the rehabilitation needs of HIV-infected children are so broad and varied, therapists need to be able to use many different approaches in treatment. They have to be flexible and adjust the treatment approach to changes in the child's health status. It is best to establish short-term goals to be revised frequently. Interventions include ongoing evaluation of the child's needs, hands-on therapy, teaching and monitoring of a home program, and adaptation of equipment.

Families need support in rehabilitation programs for children living with HIV. Most pediatric AIDS patients are eligible for Medicaid, illustrating the fact that the majority of patients come from socioeconomically impoverished families. In addition, a significant number of children live with their biological parents whereas others live with an extended family member. Approximately 10 percent of children live in foster care; thus, there is a great need for family education and support.

The rehabilitation of children with HIV infection will be affected not only by the rapidly growing numbers of patients, but also by changes in their clinical presentation in response to successful anti-retroviral treatment. Binder and Castagino (1993) concluded by stating, "Pediatric rehab professionals need to familiarize themselves with the symptoms and rehabilitation needs of HIV-infected children in order to serve them optimally." With the advent of new information in genetics and pharmacological advances, answers to some of our current questions will be provided and new questions will be formulated. Speech-language pathologists and other health care providers need to be positioned to conduct treatment efficacy research that will enhance service delivery.

The study by McNeilly (1998) further indicates the need for speech-language pathologists to monitor children born exposed to HIV who serorevert as their living environments may be a causal factor in developmental delays in the absence of HIV disease. Professionals may not know the HIV status of children as a heads up that a particular child may need to be monitored more closely than originally anticipated, based on the clinical presentation. Therefore, it is imperative that environmental and biological risk factors for all children are considered seriously, and prevention models are implemented to facilitate development.

Given that expressive and receptive language skills are particularly vulnerable to impairment based upon perinatal exposure to HIV infection, the areas of feeding, phonological, and voice problems need to be assessed. Weaknesses in these areas have been reported in children with more advanced HIV disease. Each child presents with a different profile and needs to receive an individual assessment that will result in an individually designed treatment outcome plan. The family dynamics and resources must be considered in developing a realistic optimal program for children and their families (McNeilly, 2000).

SUMMARY

This chapter provides the reader with descriptive information regarding the impact of HIV on linguistic functioning in children as well as some of the other environmental variables that also impact language development. Children with pediatric HIV exposure are a complex, heterogeneous group. Their needs vary based on medical status and environmental living conditions. As speech-language pathologists, we are cognizant of the fact that children who present with at-risk factors require early intervention to prevent or reduce the negative impact of the risk factors on their development. Go forward and effect change with effective clinical management strategies.

REFERENCES

Belman, A.L., Diamond, G., Dickson, D., Horoupian, D., Llena, J., Lantos, G., and A. Rubenstein (1998). Pediatric Acquired Immunodeficiency Syndrome: Neurologic Syndromes. *American Journal of Diseases in Children*. 142, 29-35.

Binder, H. and M. Castagnino (1993). Rehabilitation Considerations in Pediatric HIV Infection. *Physical Medicine and Rehabilitation: State of the Art Reviews*. Philadelphia: Hanley and Belfus.

Centers for Disease Control (1987). Classification System for Human Immunodeficiency Virus (HIV) Infection in Children Under 13 Years of Age. *Morbidity and Mortality Weekly Report*. 36, 225.

Centers for Disease Control (1999). HIV/AIDS Surveillance Report. 11,1. Author.

Clarren, S.K. and D.W. Smith (1978). The Fetal Alcohol Syndrome. *New England Journal of Medicine*. 298(19).1063.

Cogo. P., Laverda, A., Giaquinto, C., Zachello, F., Ades, A., Newell, M., and C. Peckham (1990). Neurological Signs in HIV Infection: Results from the European Collaborative Study. *Pediatric Infectious Disease Journal*. 9, 402-406.

Cohen, H. and G. Diamond (1992). Developmental Assessment of Children with HIV Infection. In: A.C. Crocker, H.J. Cohen, and T. Kastner, eds. *HIV Infection and Developmental Disabilities: A Resource for Service Providers*. Baltimore, MD: Brookes.

Crocker, A. (1989). Developmental Services for Children with HIV Infection. *Mental Retardation*. 27, 233.

Diamond, G.W. and H.J. Cohen (1992). Developmental Disabilities in Children with HIV Infection. In: A.C. Crocker, H.J. Cohen, and T. Kastner, eds. *HIV Infection and Developmental Disabilities: A Resource for Service Providers*. Baltimore, MD: Brookes.

Falloon, J., Eddy, J., Weiner, L., and P. Pizzo (1989). Human Immunodeficiency Virus Infection in Children. *Journal of Pediatrics*. 114(1),1-30.

Fleming, P., Gwinn, M., and M. Oxtoby (1992). Epidemiology of HIV Infection. In: R. Yogev and E. Connor, eds. *Management of HIV Infection in Infants and Children*. St Louis: Mosby-Yearbook.

Hittleman, J., Willoughby, A., Nelson, N., Gong, J. et al. (1991). Neurodevelopmental Outcome of Perinatally Acquired HIV Infection in the First 24 Months of Life [Abstract # TUB 37]. In the *Proceedings from the VII international Conference on AIDS*. 7(1), 65.

Hopkins, K.M. (1989). Emerging Patterns of Services and Case Finding for Children with HIV Infection. *Mental Retardation*. 27, 219.

Levenson, R., Kairam, R., Barnett, M., and C. Mellins (1991). Equivalence of Peabody Picture Vocabulary Test-Revised, Forms L and M for Children with Acquired Immune Deficiency Syndrome (AIDS). *Perceptual Motor Skills.* 72(1), 99-102.

Lewis, S., Reynolds-Kohler, C., Fox, H., and J. Nelson (1990). HIV-1 in Trophablastic and Villous Hofbauer Cells and Hematologic Precursors in Eight-Week Fetuses. *Lancet.* 335, 565-568.

Lifschitz, M.H., Wilson, and Smith (1985). Factors Affecting Head Growth and Intellectual Function in Children of Drug Addicts. *Pediatrics.* 75(2), 269.

McCardle, P., Nannis, E., Smith, R., and G. Fischer (1991). Patterns of Perinatal HIV-Related Language Deficit [Abstract WB 2021]. *Proceedings from the VII International Conference on AIDS. Florence, Italy.* 7(2),187.

McKinney, R. and J. Robertson (1993). Effect of Human Immunodeficiency Virus Infection on the Growth of Young Children. *Journal of Pediatrics.* 123(4), 579-582.

McNeilly, L. (1998). A Descriptive Analysis of the Receptive and Expressive Language Skills of Young Children Born to Mothers with Human Immunodeficiency Virus Infection. Doctoral dissertation. Washington, DC: Howard University.

————. (2000). Communication Intervention and Therapeutic Issues in Pediatric HIV. *Seminars in Speech and Language Vol. 21, 1.* New York: Thieme Medical Publishers.

McNeilly, L. and T. Coleman (2000). Language Disorders in Culturally Diverse Populations: Intervention Issues and Strategies. In: Coleman, T., ed. *Clinical Management of Communication Disorders in Culturally Diverse Children.* Boston, MA: Allyn and Bacon.

Meyers, A. and M. Weitzman (1991). The Newest Chronic Illness of Childhood. In: P.J. Edelson, ed. *The Pediatric Clinics of North America.* Philadelphia, PA: W.B. Saunders Co.

Noyzce, M., Diamond, G., Belma, A., Cabot, T., Douglas, C., Hopkins, K., Cohen, H., Rubinstein, A., and A. Willoughby (1989). Neurodevelopmental Impairments During Infancy in Offspring of IVDA and HIV Seropositive Mothers (Abstract). *Pediatric Research.* 25, 359A.

Pizzo, P. and C. Wilfert (eds.) (1991). *Pediatric AIDS: The Challenge of HIV Infection in Infants, Children, and Adolescents.* Baltimore, MD: Williams & Wilkins.

Pressman, H. (1992). Communication Disorders and Dysphagia in Pediatric AIDS. *ASHA.* 34, 45-47.

Rosen, T. and H. Johnson (1982). Children of Methadone-Maintained Mothers: Follow-Up to 18 Months of Age. *Journal of Pediatrics.* 101(2), 192.

Seidel, J. (1992). Psychodevelopmental Disabilities in Pediatric HIV Infection: Assessment and Intervention Strategies. University of Miami School of Medicine, FL. *International Conference on AIDS.* 8(2), B202.

Spiegel, L. and A. Mayers (1991). Psychosocial Aspects of AIDS in Children and Adolescents. In: Edelson, P.J., ed. *The Pediatric Clinics of North America.* Philadelphia, PA: W.B. Saunders Co.

Tardieu, M., Blanche, S., Duliege, A., Rouzioux, F., and C. Griscelli (1989). Neurological Involvement and Prognostic Factors after Materno-Fetal Infection [Abstract]. *Proceedings from the V International Conference on AIDS.* 1, 194.

Tardieu, M., Blanche, S.A., Rouzioux, F., Veber, F., Fisher, A., and C. Griscelli (1987). Atteintes du systeme neveux au cours des infections a HIV du nourisson. *Archieves Francais de Pediatrie.* 44, 495-499.

Watchel, R.C., Holden, W., Nair, P. et al. (1989). Neurodevelopment of Infants with Perinatally-Acquired HIV Infection. *International Conference on AIDS.* 5, 493.

Wolters, P. (1992). The Receptive and Expressive Language Functioning of Children with Acquired Immune Deficiency Syndrome. Doctoral dissertation. Chapel Hill: University of North Carolina.

Wolters, P.L., Brouwers, P., Civitello, L., and H.A. Moss (1997). Receptive and Expressive Language Function of Children with Symptomatic HIV Infection and Relationship with Disease Parameters: A Longitudinal 24-Month Follow-up Study. *AIDS.* 11(9), 1135-1144.

Wolters, P., Brouwers, P., Moss, H., and P. Pizzo (1994). The Adaptive Behavior of Children with Symptomatic HIV Infection and the Effects of AZT Therapy [Abstract # MBO.34]. *Proceedings from the XII International Conference on AIDS.* 5, 194.

Wolters, P., Brouwers, P., Moss, H., and P. Pizzo (1995). Differential Receptive and Expressive Language Functioning of Children with Symptomatic HIV Infection and Relationship with Disease Parameters: A Longitudinal 24-Month Follow-Up Study. *AIDS.* 11(9), 1135-1144.

Wolters, P., Moss, H., Eddy, J, Pizzo, P., and P. Brouwers (1989). Adaptive Behavior of Children with Symptomatic HIV Infection Before and After Zidovudine Therapy. *Journal of Pediatric Psychology.* 19, 47-61.

Ultmann, M., Belman, A., Ruff, H., Novick, B., Cone-Wesson, B., Cohen, H., and A. Rubinstein (1985). Developmental Abnormalities in Infants and Children with Acquired Immunodeficiency (AIDS) and AIDS Related complex. *Developmental Medicine and Child Neurology.* 27, 563-571.

Vohr, B. and M. Hack (1982). Developmental Follow-Up of Low-Weight Infants. *Pediatrics Clinics of North America.* 29(6),1441.

Chapter 6

Impact of Prenatal Exposure to Cocaine and Other Substances on Linguistic Functioning in Children

Lemmietta G. McNeilly

INTRODUCTION

Prenatal exposure is a significant risk factor for delayed linguistic functioning in young children. This chapter reviews the literature in this area and provides the speech-language pathologist with some concrete implications based on the reported data. Early intervention is a critical element of prevention and/or reducing the negative impact of the prenatal drug exposure on child language development.

PRENATAL DRUG EXPOSURE

Children prenatally exposed to drugs may present with a variety of profiles. Some children exhibit withdrawal symptoms, other children experience cerebral infarcts in utero, others have difficulty with stage changes, that is, movement from the state of being awake to the state of sleep.

Accumulating evidence suggests that drug abuse plays a pivotal role in the manifestation of neurodevelopmental impairments eventually seen in some children born to mothers who use drugs. Cocaine

HIV, Substance Abuse, and Communication Disorders in Children
© 2007 by The Haworth Press, Inc. All rights reserved.
doi:10.1300/5438_06

and its crack derivative have been linked to low birth weight, below average length, small head circumference, and a number of congenital malformations. Alcohol also has well-documented detrimental effects on growth, embryogenesis, and neurodevelopment. These effects range from mild fetal alcohol effects to full-blown FAS (Clarren and Smith, 1978).

The high rate of developmental abnormalities in young children with Human Immunodeficiency Virus (HIV) infection may be due to the HIV itself, or a combination of the damaging effects of illegal drugs, poor general health status, absent prenatal care and a host of environmental circumstances that can also adversely affect the developing fetus and young child (Diamond and Cohen, 1992).

LINGUISTIC FEATURES

Linguistic features of children with prenatal exposure have been studied over the past five to ten years. A review of some of this literature follows. It is difficult to isolate drug effects from other confounding variables to establish a clear causal relationship. A variety of research methodological designs have been utilized.

The 1990s presented a dramatic increase in the number of children born with prenatal exposure to cocaine. However, there is very little hard data concerning the later development of these children.

In 1993, a descriptive study conducted by Scott and colleagues (1993) at Howard University investigated the linguistic and auditory functioning of seventeen 13 to 36-month-old children at risk for speech, language, and hearing disorders due to perinatal exposure to drugs. The drugs reportedly used included cocaine, crack, marijuana, nicotine, and alcohol. Visual reinforcement audiometry and immitance were used to measure auditory functioning. Assessment of linguistic functioning was obtained from analyzing form, content, and usage of language in communication samples. In addition, auditory and linguistic results were compared with established norms.

The results of the linguistic data indicate differences in the subjects whose communication sampling was conducted in the home versus the clinic. The children seen in homes were, on average, five months younger than those children who were seen in the clinic. The number of utterances elicited in the clinic (Mean = 13.7) was far greater than the number of utterances elicited in the home (Mean = 1.4). One interpretation is that the lower number of utterances elicited in the home reflects the age of the subjects who participated rather than environmental differences. However, two of the subjects sampled at home were thirty-four months of age, which placed them in the upper end of the age range for the entire subject population. However, the differences between the language behaviors expressed by the younger group (group A) and the older children (groups B and C) were far more significant than expected. That is, the younger subjects did not utilize many opportunities to communicate and, in general, expressed very few communicative behaviors which could be analyzed. In fact, group A relied upon nonverbal communication exclusively. Reportedly, the only difference between the two groups was access to transportation and guardianship at the time of testing. The influence of the speech-language pathologist (SLP) in relation to site of sampling may also be a factor for consideration. But both sites relied upon different SLPs to elicit the samples, and all subjects participated with a SLP whom he or she had previously interacted with at least once or not at all, prior to the communication sampling.

Language form analysis revealed skills below age-level expectations. Five subjects produced simple clauses and simple clauses with adjunct expressions such as prepositional phrases and adverbs. Three of these five subjects were in the age range of 18-26 months and two were in the age range of 31-34 months. Only two of the subjects attained age expectations. Also, the entire group of subjects expressed five of Brown's fourteen morphemes. Some of the subjects expressed no morphemes (Scott et al., 1993).

Analyses of language content indicated usage of topics primarily concerned with objects expressed by subjects in groups B and C. Comments produced by groups B and C consisted primarily of nomination, some attributions, recurrence, and actions. Some of the subjects in group C also expressed spatial and possession.

In terms of phonological processes, only a few of the children exhibited age-expected simplification processes. Children between the ages of twelve and forty-eight months typically produce simplification processes. Most of the children's phonological skills were confined to productions of single vowels, bilabial, and velar phonemes. Thus, it may be concluded that these children were late in developing phonological skills, including the usage of simplification processes. Analysis of communicative intention profiles revealed that all groups of children demonstrated comments, requests for action and information, acknowledgments, responses, and protests (Scott et al., 1993).

In a study conducted by Jacobson et al. (1993), 403 black, inner-city infants born to women recruited prenatally on the basis of their alcohol consumption during pregnancy were assessed using a battery that focused on information processing and complexity of play. The results indicated that prenatal alcohol exposure was not related to visual recognition memory or cross-modal transfer of information, but was associated with longer fixation duration, a measure indicative of slower, less efficient information processing; lower scores on elicited play, and longer periods of toy exploration, possibly due to slower cognitive processing. The effects on processing speed and elicited play were dose-dependent and not attributable to maternal depression, parental intellectual stimulation, other prenatal drug exposure, or postpartum maternal drinking. The processing speed deficit is consistent with deficits in older children prenatally exposed to alcohol; this study was the first to identify slower cognitive processing in infancy and in tasks not dependent on motoric proficiency (Jacobson et al., 1993).

In an effort to assess whether children with language delays are more likely to have been exposed to cocaine in utero than children with normal language development, a case-control study was undertaken by Angelilli et al. (1994). Based on routine screening in a primary-care clinic over a one-year period, twenty-nine consecutive children were identified as language-delayed, aged twenty-four to forty-eight months. They were compared with an approximate 2:1 match of children without language delay, who had been seen in the clinic on the same days and who were of similar age. There was more reported cocaine use during pregnancy (six of twenty-nine, 21 percent) among the language-delayed children than among the controls (five of seventy-one,7 percent). This difference is statistically significant ($p < 0.05$). Discriminant analysis revealed that both cocaine and nicotine exposure were associated with delayed language development—with an unexpected negative, that is, an antagonistic, protective, interactive effect ($p < 0.005$). Neither gender nor caretaker contributed to language development in this sample. These results suggest that children with language delays, detected in a clinical setting, are more likely to have been exposed in utero to cocaine than children who exhibit normal language development. The results of this study support the claim that prenatal cocaine exposure should be considered a risk factor in monitoring development in children (Angelilli et al., 1994).

Nulman et al. (1994) conducted a case-control observational study to assess the neurodevelopment of adopted children who had been exposed in utero to cocaine. These participants included adoptive mothers and twenty-three children aged fourteen months to six-and-a-half years exposed in utero to cocaine and twenty-three age-matched control children not exposed to cocaine with their biological mothers, matched with the adoptive mothers for IQ and socioeconomic status. The setting of the study was The Hospital for Sick Children in Toronto and a consultation service for chemical exposure during pregnancy. Achievement on standard tests of cognitive and language development were among the other outcome measures utilized. The results indicated that when compared with the control group, children exposed in utero to cocaine had an eightfold increased risk for microcephaly (95 percent confidence interval 1.5 to 42.3); they also had a lower mean birth weight ($p = 0.005$) and a lower gestational age ($p = 0.002$). In follow-up, the cocaine-exposed children caught up with the control subjects in weight and stature but not in head circumference (mean 31st percentile versus 63rd percentile) ($p = 0.001$). Although there were no significant differences between the two groups in global IQ, the cocaine-exposed children had significantly lower scores than the control subjects on the Reynell language test for both verbal comprehension ($p = 0.003$) and expressive language ($p = 0.001$). Reportedly, this was the first study to document that intrauterine exposure to cocaine is associated with measurable and clinically significant toxic neurologic effects, independent of postnatal home and environmental cofounders. Because women who use cocaine during pregnancy almost invariably smoke cigarettes and often use alcohol, it is impossible to attribute the measured toxic effects to cocaine alone (Nulman et al., 1994).

Hawley et al. (1995) conducted a study to compare the cognitive, language, and emotional development of twenty cocaine-exposed preschool children and with the developmental skills of twenty-four noncocaine-exposed children. Group differences were notably significant in emotional and behavioral status. Maternal report was utilized to assess these skills; however, few differences in cognitive and language development were actually obtained (Hawley et al., 1995).

Mentis and Lundgren (1995) conducted a preliminary study to compare the language development profiles of five children prenatally exposed to cocaine and associated risk factors to the language development profiles of a matched nonexposed control group. The discourse-pragmatic, semantic, and form components of language analyses were utilized. The language evaluation was based on the analysis of a thirty-minute language sample. The results suggested differences between the two groups as well as differences within the cocaine-exposed group. The major differences between the two groups were in discourse-pragmatics although less marked differences in syntactic development were also found. The results of this study suggest that children with prenatal exposure to cocaine in combination with multiple associated risk factors may exhibit compromised language development (Mentis and Lundgren, 1995).

Bender and colleagues (1995) explored the developmental correlates of prenatal and/or postnatal crack-cocaine exposure in children between four and six years of age. Three groups were studied. Group 1 consisted of eighteen prenatally exposed children whose mothers continue to use crack. Group II was composed of twenty-eight children without prenatal exposure whose mothers presently use crack. Group III comprised twenty-eight children whose mothers never used crack. Mothers were street-recruited and were comparable in race and socioeconomic status. The three groups of children did not differ on neurological, gross motor, or expressive language measures. However, prenatally exposed children performed significantly worse than the other subjects on receptive language and visual motor drawing tests (Bender et al., 1995).

A prospective longitudinal study on the development of children of drug-dependent mothers who used combinations of cocaine, heroin, and methadone during pregnancy was carried out in Amsterdam by Van-Baar and De-Graaff (1994). The children and a contrast reference group were followed from birth to 5 1/2, 4, 4 1/2 and 5 1/2 years. The children of drug-dependent mothers repeatedly showed delays in cognitive functioning at preschool-age. Individual difficulties, as well as differences in developmental patterns over time, were found most clearly when facets of language development formed part of the assessments. Van-Baar concludes that early intervention programs should focus on enhancement of communication, in addition to the children's ability to adapt to task situation (Van-Baar and De-Graaff, 1994).

A significant number of children are born to women who consume drugs such as alcohol, cocaine, heroin, methadone, marijuana, and/or phencyclidine (PCP) during pregnancy. As a result, some children exhibit both physical and developmental delays. It has been reported that children with FAS have growth problems, attention deficit disorders, and other medical issues. Impaired cognitive and neurologic functioning through the first two years of life has been documented for children exposed to methadone while in utero. Those children exposed to polydrug use, including cocaine and marijuana, seem to have difficulties with language development and verbal skills. Some of these deficiencies show improvement with early intervention and a nurturing environment, but in many cases the impairment continues throughout childhood (D'Apolito-K, 1998).

Findings from a study conducted by Koren and colleagues (1998) indicate that children exposed in utero to cocaine are at risk for long-term neurobehavioral damage, not just because of the drug itself, but also because of clustering of other health determinants. These include low socioeconomic status, low maternal education, and maternal addiction. Koren further suggests that one methodologic approach to separate the direct neurotoxic effects of cocaine from these synergistic insults is to conduct a follow-up study of a cohort of children exposed in utero to cocaine and given up for adoption to middle- and upper-class families. The Toronto Adoption study, supported by Health Canada, has proven the direct neurotoxic effects of cocaine on IQ and language. These effects are mild to moderate as compared to those measured in children exposed in utero to cocaine and reared by their natural mothers (Koren et al., 1998).

IMPLICATIONS FOR SLPs

Based on the diverse findings of studies conducted with children prenatally exposed to cocaine and other drugs, an array of implications are significant for SLPs working with pediatric populations. Many of the groups of children studied exhibited delays in language acquisition, phonological processes, attention, and processing information. The findings are inconclusive regarding how much prenatal exposure determines the extent to which linguistic delays or disorders may result. It is important to note that all children with prenatal drug exposure do not exhibit linguistic delays or disorders. However, a significant number of children do exhibit communication deficits, especially during the first two years of life.

The complexity of sensory and attentional deficits, paired with linguistic and cognitive impairments, can make intervention planning a challenge. It is also efficacious for SLPs to work collaboratively with other health care professionals. Co-treatments with occupational therapists and physical therapists can increase performance levels significantly. Frequent ongoing two-way communication with parent and other professionals involved in management is also imperative for successful attainment of targeted goals. It may be necessary to change the schedule of speech therapy sessions to follow occupational or physical therapy to maximize the child's feeding/swallowing, and oral motor skills should be conducted to rule out any problems. Undiagnosed problems in these areas could lead to long-term problems and difficulties in phonological development. Prioritization of goals should be mutually agreed upon by families and professionals involved in therapeutic intervention for the child.

SUMMARY

Based upon the results of the various studies that have investigated communication skills of children with prenatal drug exposure, it can be concluded that varied outcomes may range from normally developing skills to severe delays, which may be manifested across multiple skill areas, that is, motor, attention, language, and cognition. Early intervention is important and should include periodic screenings of communication and audiological skills, since many children present with recurrent otitis media, which impacts acquisition of language.

Children who receive early intervention exhibit a reduction in delays or present with no developmental delays. Routine developmental monitoring facilitates the early identification of problems and the implementation of early intervention. As SLPs involved in screenings of young children, we may be among the first professionals to identify a delay and/or recommend services to families.

Living environments also contribute to skill acquisition in all children. When a child lives in a drug-seeking culture and the primary caregiver actively uses a variety of substances, children are at an increased environmental risk for developmental delays. Children born with biological risk factors caused by the prenatal drug exposure are at even greater risk for developmental delays when they also have to contend with environmental risk factors. It is important that social workers, physicians, early interventionists, and SLPs collaborate to enroll children into early intervention programs.

It is important to keep in mind that children born with prenatal drug exposure are a heterogeneous group. These children also often make significant gains developmentally when their development is monitored periodically to identify delays. Furthermore, these children also make satisfactory progress with enrollment in early intervention programs designed to address their identified weaknesses. Parental involvement and education regarding normal development and communication/feeding facilitation skills also greatly enhance these children's opportunities to be ready for kindergarten. Finally, it is important that we refrain from stereotyping children based on prenatal histories. These children can and do learn, given appropriate opportunities.

REFERENCES

Angelilli, M., Fischer, H., Delaney-Black, V., Rubenstein, M., Ager, J., and R. Sokol. History of In Utero Cocaine Exposure in Language-Delayed Children. *Clinical Pediatrics*. September 1994; 33(9), 514-516.

Bender, S., Word, C., DiClemente, R., Crittenden, M., Persuad, N., and L. Ponton. The Developmental Implications of Prenatal and/or Postnatal Crack Cocaine Exposure in Preschool Children: A Preliminary Report. *Journal of Developmental Behavior in Pediatrics*. December 1995; 16(6), 418-424; discussion 425-430.

Clarren, S.K. and D.W. Smith. The Fetal Alcohol Syndrome. *New England Journal of Medicine*. 1978; 298(19),1063.

D'Apolito, K. Substance Abuse: Infant and Childhood Outcomes. *Journal of Pediatric Nursing*. October 1998; 13(5), 307-316.

Diamond, G.W. and H.J. Cohen (1992). Developmental Disabilities in Children with HIV Infection. In: A.C. Crocker, H.J. Cohen, and T. Kastner, eds. *HIV In-*

fection and Developmental Disabilities: A Resource for Service Providers. Baltimore, MD: Brookes.

Hawley, T., Halle, T., Drasin, R., and N. Thomas. Children of Addicted Mothers: Effects of the "Crack Epidemic" on the Caregiving Environment and the Development of Preschoolers. *American Journal of Orthopsychiatry.* July 1995; 65(3), 364-379.

Jacobson, S., Jacobson, J., Sokol, R., Martier, S., and Ager, J. Prenatal Alcohol Exposure and Infant Information Processing Ability. *Child Development.* December 1993; 64(6), 1706-1721.

Koren, G., Nulman, I., Rovet, J., Greenbaum, R., Loebstein, M., and T. Einarson. Long-Term Neurodevelopmental Risks in Children Exposed In Utero to Cocaine. The Toronto Adoption Study. *Annals of New York Academic Science.* June 21, 1998; 846, 306-313.

Mentis, M. and Lundgren, K. Effects of Prenatal Exposure to Cocaine and Associated Risk Factors on Language Development. *Journal of Speech and Hearing Research.* December 1995; 38(6), 1303-1318.

Nulman, I., Rovet, J., Altmann, D., Bradley, C., Einarson, T., and G. Koren. Neurodevelopment of Adopted Children Exposed In Utero to Cocaine. *CMAJ.* December 1, 1994; 151(11), 1591-1597.

Scott, D., Lee-Wilkerson, D., McNeilly, L., and S. Gray. A Descriptive Analysis of Auditory and Linguistic Skills Exhibited by Children with Perinatal Drug Exposure. *ECHO.* February 1993.

Van-Baar, A. and B. De-Graaff. Cognitive Development at Preschool-Age of Infants of Drug-Dependent Mothers. *Developmental Medicine in Child Neurology.* December 1994; 36(12), 1063-1075.

Chapter 7

Effects of Cocaine
on the Human Nervous System

In the 1980s, cocaine was considered an "emblem of the slim and fashionable . . . [and] in 1985 the United States reported 5.7 million users" (Dajer, 1998). Since that time, the number of people who reportedly use this illicit substance have dropped by over half, but the numbers are rising once again. For the first time since 1985, among high school seniors, the use of cocaine is rising, from 9 percent in 1995 to 12.6 percent in 1997 (Dajer, 1998). For women of the child-bearing age group, eighteen to twenty-five years old, 22.2 percent of white women, 21.2 percent of black women, and 15.4 percent of Hispanic women said they have used drug (Sparks, 1993). There are approximately 2 million people who use cocaine. However, the amount of research that has been done on the effects of cocaine, especially to the brain, has been minimal (Di Sclafani and Trura, 1998). An important finding of some of the statistics stated earlier is that illegal drug use is not just a problem of minorities in the inner cities. Statistically, more whites use drugs, especially those located in rural and suburban America (Sparks, 1993).

Cocaine is a powdery, white substance that is a CNS stimulator. It is made from the leaves of the coca bush, specifically erythroxylon coca. When this substance is ingested, one gets a "feeling of extreme well-being" that lasts a half hour or less (Dajer, 1998). Throughout history, natives in the Andes Mountains in South America have used this substance for its strengthening properties, and here in America, it was used as a main ingredient in medicines and tonics. Even by the

HIV, Substance Abuse, and Communication Disorders in Children
© 2007 by The Haworth Press, Inc. All rights reserved.
doi:10.1300/5438_07

beginning of the twentieth century, cocaine was recognized as an addictive substance that could compromise one's health. However, it was not until two professional athletes died within ten days of each other in June of 1986 that the public began to open its eyes to the dangers of cocaine use.

EFFECTS UPON THE HUMAN BODY

Cocaine use has many negative side effects on the body. It takes about three-seven years of inhaling this drug to develop a severe addiction to it, but its effects can be felt immediately. Symptoms of cocaine use include, profuse sweating, fixed and dilated pupils, decreased appetite, a runny nose, increased heart rate and blood pressure, an indifference to pain and fatigue, a constriction of blood vessels, a numbing of the mucous membranes in the nose, throat, and mouth, restlessness, a sore throat, chest pain, shortness of breath, and mood swings. With prolonged use the nasal septum will deteriorate. One may also experience depression, insomnia, weight loss, and heart strain. "Seizures are a frequent complication of cocaine use and can occur after a single dose" (Di Sclafani and Trura, 1998). In addition, the addict may experience cocaine psychosis, which includes the idea that bugs are crawling under one's skin, along with possible tremors, paranoia, and hallucinations. Furthermore, cocaine has a negative effect on the immune system. Cocaine addicts have an increased risk of contracting hepatitis, HIV, and endocarditis, and an inflammation of the lining of the heart and heart valves.

EFFECTS UPON THE BRAIN

Cocaine has major effects on the brain. When ingested it moves to nerve synapses in the deep portions of the brain. This area of the brain houses regions that are associated with the feelings of pleasure and reward. Here the drug increases the activity of the neurotransmitters, dopamine, and norepinephrine. Normally these chemicals are released by the brain to perform their duty and then they are reabsorbed. Cocaine prevents this reuptake of the chemicals by blocking nerve endings and, therefore, allowing the neurotransmitters to act for longer periods of time than is normal. It has also been found to bind to the basal ganglia, and if the cocaine is smoked as crack, there is an even faster absorption of the drug and high brain concentrations of the cocaine.

Cocaine's major effects on the brain have many lasting side effects. Cocaine has been associated with cognitive and sensory distortions as well as learning memory alterations. The blood vessels of the brain become extremely constricted when using cocaine. The blood vessels can become so constricted that the brain fails to get any blood, resulting in a stroke. This constriction of cerebral arteries can lead to cognitive dysfunction. Complications in cocaine-exposed infants can include a grade III intraventricular hemorrhaging, which may cause severe brain damage that results in cerebral palsy.

Research has shown that cerebral vasoconstriction occurs approximately twenty minutes after cocaine use. This vasoconstriction probably occurs because of an increase in serotonin, which is the most potent vasoconstrictor (Zegans and Temoshok, 1990). In addition, those subjects who received higher doses of the drug were more likely to experience this constriction. Prior cocaine usage may cause a cumulative effect on the constriction of the cerebral arteries, as shown by a study performed at McLean Hospital in Belmont, Massachusetts. Subjects in this study who had used cocaine in larger amounts in the past experienced a greater narrowing of the cerebral arteries (Stocker, 1998).

It has also been found that cocaine addicts who are drug free for three-five weeks are "impaired in most measures of learning and explicit memory, but normal in measures of sustained attention" (Di Sclafani and Trura, 1998). This is because "cocaine could cause persistent blood flow deficits in the brain" that persist after use is discontinued (Stocker, 1998). Those addicts who were "clean" for longer periods of time continued to show problems in retaining nonverbal information. Problems with memory may occur because of functional or neurochemical abnormalities in the hippocampus. They may also occur because of abnormalities in other areas of the brain, like the frontal cortex, resulting from deficient input and output from the hippocampus. Such abnormalities have been found through computerized axial tomography scans (CT scans). These scans have demonstrated "morphological changes in patients who developed neurological symptoms after cocaine consumption" (Di Sclafani and Trura, 1998). Such cerebral pathology also is associated with subarachnoid hemorrhages, intracerebral hemorrhages, and cerebral infarction (the dying brain tissue).

The previously mentioned effects on the brain can have a major impact on an individual's speech and language. If someone experiences a stroke because of the constriction of cerebral arteries, then there is always the possibility of aphasia. Aphasia is a loss of language, which can range in severity. Loss of blood supply to areas of the brain could affect important language areas, causing a variety of language and learning problems. Anytime blood flow is kept from a portion of the human body, there is the possibility that the tissue dies. If brain tissue dies, it cannot be regenerated.

EFFECTS UPON THE HEART

Cocaine abusers have also been found "to have enlarged hearts and thickened cardiac muscles" (Gold, 1993). These cocaine users found with such symptoms are people who never previously had a history of these problems. In addition, cocaine use can cause the left ventricle of the heart to hypertrophy, which leads to an increased risk of arrythmias, sudden death, and strokes. These are only a few of the effects that this drug can have on the cardiovascular system, for cocaine has been "linked to every type of heart disease" (Gold, 1993).

EFFECTS UPON SPEECH AND LANGUAGE

The heart is the organ that is responsible for pumping blood to all parts of the body. If this does not happen, death results. Speech structures are affected by this because they too require blood supply. If they are not provided with an adequate blood supply, they will deteriorate and will not be able to be used in aiding the production of speech.

Lastly, cocaine abuse also affects the respiratory system. It depresses the respiratory system and increases the risk of pulmonary infection. Cocaine suppresses the transport of mucus in the respiratory tract. Black or bloody sputum (saliva that is mixed with mucus that is released from the lungs or respiratory passages) can be brought up by individuals. Taking cocaine by freebasing or smoking can alter the way in which gas is exchanged by the lungs and pulmonary function overall. This ingestion irritates both small and large airways. Cocaine has been known to cause such problems as brochospasms, lung damage, pulmonary edema, nosebleeds, and sinusitis.

Cocaine use can result in respiratory failure, which in turn causes sudden death. This respiratory failure can result from a "cocaine induced inhibition of medullary centers in the brain" (Gold, 1993). However, it can also impact someone's life in a less severe way that is just as important. When people speak, they are utilizing their breath stream in such a way that the vocal folds are forced into movement. This is one of the first steps in speech production. If pulmonary function is altered or inhibited, it will alter one's speech patterns. The ability to speak may be lost completely. The air resulting respiration is not only used for biological functions, but also for speaking. Someone's ability to communicate can be severely curbed, leading to the need for alternate forms of communication, like augmentative communication.

PREGNANCY AND COCAINE USE

There is a rapidly growing body of research strongly suggesting that prenatal substance is linked to health problems in a child's development. No reliable national estimate of the extent or patterns of cocaine use during pregnancy exist. However, in 1991, Gomby and Shiono estimated that between 554,400 and 739,200 infants each year may be exposed in utero to one or more illicit drugs. Depending on the population studied and the method used, prevalence estimates from individual hospitals range from 3 to 50 percent of live births. Higher incidents are most often reported from centers serving poor, inner-city mothers (Sparks, 1993). A study done in Florida stated that despite similar rates of substance abuse among black and white women, black women were tested and reported at approximately ten times the rate for white women, and poor women were more likely to be reported (Sparks, 1993). It has been concluded that the use of illicit drugs is common among pregnant women, regardless of race and socioeconomic status.

When females are pregnant and taking cocaine, they often do not think of the impact this will have upon their unborn child. Cocaine use restricts blood flow to the fetus when uterine, placental, and umbilical blood vessels constrict. This constriction causes a decreased nutrient and gas exchange between mother and fetus. This retards the fetus' growth. If this constriction occurs during critical growth periods, it causes congenital malformations.

Being exposed to such conditions in utero can be extremely detrimental to a child. Many fetuses do not even survive long enough to be born. Those who are live births have decreased birth weight, small head circumference, growth retardation, and neurobehavioral deficits. These infants are also often premature. As these children grow, they often have behavioral and learning difficulties. They cannot sit long enough to focus in order to learn. They may exhibit problems acquiring language and be presented with lifelong delays in language, learning, and social skills.

Furthermore, neurobehavioral patterns of cocaine-exposed infants can be divided into two extreme behaviors: excitable and depressed. These two behavior patterns are due to the direct and indirect effects of cocaine. Researchers have described excitable children as easily aroused infants exhibiting irritability, excessive and high-pitched cry, tremors, nervousness, and hypertonicity. Depressed infants are underaroused, difficult to wake, have fleeting attention, and low control of orientation. In addition to these two behavioral patterns, there are other neurobehavioral risks of prenatal cocaine exposure in infancy. These risks include deficiencies in interactive abilities, seizures, hipotonicity, and hyperactivity (Sparks, 1993).

Based on research, it appears that cocaine-exposed infants have behaviors in specific areas that may affect differentiating behaviors in the areas of cognitive orientation involving visual and auditory response, and motor development, involving muscle tone (Sparks, 1993).

A majority of these children produce nonverbal speech. Their intonation patterns are like those of normal speech, but their words are unintelligible. Researchers also state that children exposed to cocaine have an increased difficulty with verbal and nonverbal reasoning. These children also have more difficulty with sound discrimination, prefer easier tasks, and give up on tasks early. Furthermore, articulation problems are evident, but do not differ significantly from those unexposed children in similar environments. Cocaine-exposed children do not prosper in a distracted learning environment. They usually become socially withdrawn or very violent. These children also tend to develop audiological manifestations of their early drug exposure (Sparks, 1993).

Some infants who are exposed to cocaine exhibit common oral-motor behaviors. Some of these behaviors include a poor suck/swallow pattern, poor tongue stabilization in midline, tongue thrust, and tongue tremors. These behaviors can affect and inhibit the correct sound production, articulation, and intelligibility of speech.

Moreover, it appears that prenatal drug exposure does have predictable adverse effects on developmental processes that extend beyond the infancy period in many children. Some of these long-term effects are having reduced self-regulation, being easily distracted, using less representational play, and having attachment problems. These long-term effects lead to an important inference for SLPs. Since a link between representational play and language acquisition has been demonstrated, SLPs can anticipate a risk of problems in language development for drug-exposed children at later ages.

CONCLUSION

Cocaine is a devastating drug that impacts our society greatly. This drug not only affects adults but is now beginning to affect our life line of this world—infants. We can make a difference with drug-exposed children by helping their parents, and by providing appropriate early intervention.

The side effects, mentioned earlier, of using cocaine are extremely important issues and need to be addressed. Every day, many people are causing themselves detrimental harm because they are hooked on cocaine and may lack the resources (family, friends, money, information, medical access, etc.) to kick the habit. Addicts may also choose not to seek help. If resources are more readily available and treatment options are publicized and discussed, the problem of cocaine use and abuse may decrease. Individuals need to be made aware that there are other ways to feel good, to fill the void in their lives, and to deal with all of life's stresses without taking drugs. The consumption of drugs affects more than just the user. Society as a whole continues to lose if drug addiction and its effects are not fully addressed. The biggest losers will be the children, who are directly affected by this drug use.

REFERENCES

Dajer, Tony (1998). Snowed. *Discover.* 19, 40-47.

Di Sclafani, Victoria and Diana Trura (1998). Abstinent Chronic Crack-Cocaine and Crack-Cocaine/Alcohol Abusers Evidence Normal Hippocampal Volumes on MRI Despite Persistent Cognitive Impairments. *Addiction Biology.* 3, 261-268.

Gold, Mark S. (1993). *Drugs of Abuse: A Comprehensive Series for Clinicians-Cocaine.* Vol. 3. New York: Plenum Medical Book Company.

Sparks, Shirley N. (1993). *Children of Prenatal Substance Abuse: School Age Children.* San Diego, CA: Singular Publishing.

Stocker, Steven. NIDA NOTES—Cocaine Abuse May Lead to Strokes and Mental Deficits. http://165.112.78.61/NIDA_Notes/NNVol13N3/Xcocaine.html, October 5, 1998, 8:31 p.m.

Zegans, L. and Temoshok, Lydia (1990). *Cocaine in the Brain.* New Brunswick: Rutgers University Press.

Chapter 8

Fetal Alcohol Syndrome (FAS) and Language Disorders

For centuries people have theorized that alcohol consumption during pregnancy has adverse effects on the fetus. Lemonine et al. (1968) verified in their study that children of alcoholic women may be harmed by the prenatal exposure. During the past decade, there has been a dramatic increase in the number of children born with prenatal exposure to alcohol. FAS results from excessive prenatal exposure to alcohol. FAS is a pattern of altered tissue and organ development that involves cardiovascular problems, head and facial abnormalities such as a flattened mid-face, a small jaw, and a thin upper lip; prenatal growth deficiency with developmental delays; and CNS dysfunctions causing intellectual impairment. The head and facial abnormalities usually result in a cleft palate. FAS children are typically under the third percentile in height, weight, and head circumference (Kinsley, 1991). A variety of CNS (defined as the brain and spinal cord) deficits results from FAS, including mild to moderate retardation. These children will also have a subaverage IQ and poor self-help skills. Few FAS children have normal intelligence and most are significantly handicapped (Kinsley, 1991). Reported communication problems include delayed language and problems with speech articulation, fluency, and swallowing. A language delay is defined as the child learning in an appropriate sequence but doing it at a slower rate with acceptable errors, while articulation problems include the inability to produce speech sounds properly.

Children with FAS may have no visible effects and may just have subclinical FAS, also known as a FAE, and, therefore, go untreated.

HIV, Substance Abuse, and Communication Disorders in Children
© 2007 by The Haworth Press, Inc. All rights reserved.
doi:10.1300/5438_08

Subclinical FAS is a subtle version of FAS, with hidden defects including learning disabilities. Subclinical FAS refers to a heterogeneous group of disorders with difficulty in acquisition and use of listening, reading, writing, speaking, and mathematical abilities. In general, longitudinal studies of the effects of prenatal exposure to alcohol on the CNS indicate that alcohol-exposed children do less well on developmental tests, have deficits on IQ testing, and exhibit signs of problematic behavior, including inattention and hyperactivity (Day, 1992). It is important to study these children because they have created a new population of language disorders. They suffer from abnormal acquisition, comprehension, or expression of spoken or written language. FAS is a leading cause of birth defects characterized by mental retardation.

In the United States, one to three children born out of every 1,000 births have some degree of FAS. Therefore, FAS is the leading cause of mental retardation in the modern Western world today. Between two and ten times as many people suffer some effect of alcohol exposure, even though they do not exhibit the full FAS. If these statistics are correct, between 2,000 and 12,000 of the projected 14 million children born in the United States each year will demonstrate some effects of FAS/E.

Some studies have shown that alcohol use, even at levels of less than a drink per day, can affect growth and development. Larroque et al. report that they detected effects on the development of the fetus' CNS at maternal intake levels of three or more drinks per day (Larroque et al., 1995).

Researchers Bach and Wasson have studied the multiple aspects of FAS and direct effects they have on children. Approximately one-fifth of patients surveyed had some degree of a hearing loss due to alcohol exposure (Bach and Wasson, 1991). Their research revealed that all of the patients had some degree of articulation disorder. Bach and Wasson found their surveys that the patients displayed a range of voice disorders, including breathiness, harsh/hoarsened voice, increased pitch, increased intensity, monotone, and decreased intensity. Approximately 11.7 percent of the patients with FAS exhibited some type of fluency disorder (Bach and Wasson, 1991). Bach and Wasson's studies also revealed that most patients with FAS showed both receptive-and expressive-language disorders. Morphologic/syntactic disorders, semantic disorders, and pragmatic disorders occurred at an approximate frequency of 10-20 percent.

Larroque et al. (1995) studied moderate prenatal alcohol exposure and psychomotor development at the preschool age. Their study focused on the psychomotor development of preschool-age children in a population that included a high proportion of mothers who drank various quantities of alcohol and who did not consume illicit drugs. Children of mothers who consumed 1.5 oz of absolute alcohol or more per day during pregnancy had poor psychomotor development (Larroque et al., 1995). This study showed that moderate to heavy alcohol consumption during pregnancy, at levels well below those associated with FAS, had effects on children's psychomotor development. Day et al. (1992) studied prenatal exposure to alcohol and its effect on infant growth and morphologic characteristics. An increased risk of having a low birth weight baby was associated with alcohol consumption in the first and/or second month of pregnancy. Maternal drinking during the early first trimester was also associated with an increased risk of giving birth to an infant who was below the 10th percentile for length or head circumference, or who had either a minor physical anomaly or fetal alcohol effect. The use of alcohol in the first and/or second month of pregnancy was significantly associated with reduced head circumference of the neonate. Alcohol consumption in previous studies was associated with an increased risk of low birth weight, length, and head circumference below the 10th percentile. Factors that cause growth retardation early in pregnancy, in general, affect all of the growth parameters equally (Day et al., 1992).

With regard to language development, only a few studies have been reported. Although the results are inconclusive, they do suggest that language is vulnerable to disruption due to the effects of alcohol on cognitive development. That data to date suggest that infants with prenatal alcohol exposure demonstrated impaired fetal growth, altered behavior as newborns, and CNS damage. This suggests that prenatal alcohol exposure and associated risk factors may place children at risk for later cognitive and language development.

Nearly every study on FAS or FAE, regardless of client age, reports a discrepancy between subject ability to use verbal language and ability to communicate effectively (Abkarian, 1992). Becker et al. (1990) did a quantitative and qualitative comparison of FAS and normal subjects. This study showed that, qualitatively, the FAS subjects did not produce as syntactically complex grammatical structures as did younger normals, nor did they produce appropriate responses in dialogue when compared to younger normal children. When compared with children of similar age and mental ability, qualitative differences in performance were exhibited. Variability in performance was manifested more often in language production rather than in language comprehension tasks.

Hamilton (1981) and Becker et al. (1990) researched the language and speech abilities of children with FAS. They reported uneven language performances among their subjects. In some areas, subjects were not significantly different from controls matched by MLU or nonverbal cognitive ability.

In summary, research comparing the speech and language abilities of FAS children with those of normal children has shown the following (Becker, Warr-Leeper, and Leeper, 1990):

Grammatical Abilities

1. The FAS children did not demonstrate comprehension of morphological and syntactic forms for picture identification to the same degree as the younger controls.
2. The FAS children produced fewer grammatically accurate and complete sentences in spontaneous conversation when compared to the younger controls.
3. The FAS children did not demonstrate comprehension of verbal commands to the same degree as their younger controls.

Semantic Abilities. The FAS children did not demonstrate comprehension of single word vocabulary to the same degree as younger controls.

Memory Abilities. The FAS children demonstrated poorer ability to store linguistic elements in short-term memory when compared to younger controls.

Articulation Abilities. The FAS subjects more often demonstrated severe impairments in the production of speech sounds than did controls matched for nonverbal cognitive ability.

FAS AMONG NATIVE AMERICANS

Women who drink heavily during pregnancy run a 50 percent risk if harming the fetus. One-third of children born to alcoholic drinkers will have FAS; of moderate drinkers FAS will occur at about a rate of 10 percent. Twenty-three percent of white women drink during pregnancy in comparison to 16 percent of black women and 9 percent of Mexican-American women. Studies have shown that there are certain groups of women who are likely to give birth to children who will have FAS. The remarkable truth is that women who fall in the following group(s) are more likely to have FAS/E children: women who are college educated, unmarried women, female students, women who smoke, and women in households with $50,000 or greater income (Kellerman, www.fas.htm).

An even sadder truth is that alcohol abuse is even worse on Indian reservations where FAS has been reported in 1 in every 100 children (Streissguth, 1997). Among Native Americans, the incidence varies between the cultures. Clinicians servicing the Navajo and Pueblo tribes report FAS rates similar to that for the overall U.S. population, while for the Indians in the Southwest Plains a much higher prevalence is reported. In one very small Native American community, the incidence of FAS has reached as high as one in every eight live births (Streissguth, 1997). FAS has reached catastrophic levels among Native American communities. At this rate FAS has the ability to demolish Native American cultures in only a few generations.

Native Americans are attempting to band together to educate themselves and fight FAS. The Seventh Generation Fetal Alcohol Syndrome Prevention Project is being instituted among Native American communities nationwide (7th Generation Project). The "7th Generation" is indicative of and ignites emotions common to all Nations of Indian people. The "7th Generation" refers to responsibility to and for Mother Earth and responsibility to and for future generations. Tribal leaders and elders teach that each seventh generation is responsible for the survival of the people until the following seventh generation. Native American leaders are teaching that it is now the time of the seventh generation, and it is time to assume responsibility to ensure that present and future generations may live well.

The American Indian Institute has developed a learning module for presentation to classrooms for native students in the sixth, seventh, and eighth grades (Ma, 1998). They are currently creating learning modules complete with videotapes and curriculum guides for Native American high school students as well. These prevention efforts will receive national recognition for the fight against FAS. This information will be welcomed by school systems. In a study published in the *Journal of School Health* in 1998, Native Americans in the sixth through eight grades were surveyed about their attitudes and their knowledge of the risk factors and prevention strategies associated with FAS (Ma, 1998). Studies show that 52 percent of the students had partaken of alcohol prior to the survey. Even though many were sexually active, they lacked knowledge about the relationship between alcohol and FAS (Ma, 1998).

In the middle 1980s, a group of Native Americans living on and in the surrounding area of the Yankton Sioux Reservation in South Dakota formed the Native American Community Board (NACB). The first NACB project was "Women and Children in Alcohol: A Fetal Alcohol Syndrome Program." This nonprofit organization has received political recognition and is making moves to educate young people, and especially young women. The NACB founded the Native American Women's Health Education Resource Center, which concentrates on alcohol and domestic violence issues.

The hospitals that assist higher populations of Native Americans are also concerned with the huge influx of children born with FAS. These hospitals are attempting to detect which children could be at risk of having FAS for the best possible outcome of the child. In a 1998 study by the Aberdeen Area Indian Health Service at PHS Indian Hospital in South Dakota, researchers were concerned with the detection of alcohol use in the prenatal population (on a Northern Plains Reservation) using various methods. Reports have shown that FAS is markedly high among American Indian populations (Gale, White, and Welty, 1998). Unfortunately, no screening toil has been validated to measure or show alcohol use in American Indian Women. Researchers concentrated on self-administered questionnaires and hospital records to determine any history of alcohol-related illnesses or injuries as a means of comparison with the results of the questionnaire. The study showed that between 20 and 71 percent drank alcohol during their pregnancy (Gale, White, and Welty, 1998). As a result of the large variation, the clinicians are able to reevaluate their previous screening methods and are now concocting better methods and specific questions written for the target population.

Alcohol is a teratogenic agent that causes defects in the developing embryo and fetus. Language deficits due to CNS damage or dysfunction are also evident in the FAS individual. There is only limited information regarding the language deficits associated with FAS among the American Indian population. The TOLD-P and the TOLD-I were administered by SLPs to twenty-seven American-Indian children (Carney, 1991). Ten of the children had FAS and seventeen were normally developing control subjects. Research showed that the younger FAS children demonstrated global language deficits while the older FAS children exhibited syntactic deficits (Carney and Chermak, 1991).

FAS is associated with four kinds of hearing disorders: developmentally delayed auditory function, sensorineural hearing loss (Church and Abel, 1998). As a result of craniofacial anomalies and hearing impairments, speech and language pathologies are common in FAS patients. Individuals with FAS who have craniofacial anomalies will also probably be mentally retarded and suffer from multiple hearing problems. These confounded defects will especially impact upon articulation and phonological development.

Hearing disorders are a form of sensory deprivation. If this is present during early childhood, the result is permanent hearing, language, and mental impairment. Early identification and intervention to treat hearing, language, and speech disorders could mean an improved outcome for the FAS child. Formal communication skills assessments were successfully completed on eight children validly diagnosed with forms of FAS. The subjects ranged in ages from four and a half to nine and a half years. All of the FAS children, except for one, expressed abnormalities in the speech mechanism within at least one of the major valves along the vocal tract (Becker, Warr-Leeper, and Leeper, 1990). In three of the FAS children, when matched for nonverbal cognitive ability, inconsistent mental age articulation abilities were found. The FAS children also demonstrated mental age inconsistent abilities in the comprehension and use of grammatical markers, both in repetition and in spontaneous language tasks (Becker, Warr-Leeper, and, Leeper, 1990). When compared to non-FAS children the

FAS subjects exhibited reduced capacity to process and store critical elements (Becker, Warr-Leeper, and Leeper, 1990).

The congenital anomalies expressed by persons with FAS are traditionally associated with hearing disorders. In a study conducted at Wayne State University School of Medicine, results showed that 77 percent of FAS patients suffer from intermittent conductive hearing loss due to recurrent otitis media that began early in childhood and persisted into adulthood (Gale, White, and Welty, 1998). Native Americans tend to have higher rates of otitis media. The literature is unclear whether higher rates of otitis media are due to poverty on Indian reservations or whether Native Americans are predisposed to succumb to this infection. Twenty-seven percent have sensorineural hearing loss in addition to the conductive hearing loss. It appears that everyone who suffers from FAS has significantly impaired central hearing function. Even mild, intermittent hearing loss due to middle ear infections can adversely affect language and speech acquisition, which later negatively impacts academic achievement. In general, the greater the hearing loss, the more impaired the speech signal that may be heard, but because of the hearing loss, it may be distorted and, therefore, inaccurately decoded. Adequate auditory sensitivity is crucial for normal language acquisition and development in children. Ninety percent of individuals suffering from FAS have some sort of speech deficit and 76 percent have expressive language deficits. Hearing, speech, and language deficits among this population do not appear to be influenced by age.

The neurologic impairments and cognitive deficits demonstrated by persons with FAS cannot be fully explained by generally lower IQ scores (Church and Abel, 1998). Even the nonretarded FAS patients commonly exhibit behavior problems, decreased social competence, and poor school performance. Native Americans generally live in poverty-stricken areas. Poverty alone can cause CNS damage because babies born in poorer areas are more likely to have low birth weight. Pair propensity for CNS damage with FAS and the child will suffer from long-term language problems so debilitating that he will be unable to recover. The CNS damage sustained during prenatal development will facilitate problems with pragmatic abilities. Deficits were also noted on attentional and memory tasks tapping visual-spatial skills, declarative learning, and cognitive flexibility and planning

(Church and Abel, 1998). FAS patients also demonstrated difficulties in processing speed, accuracy, and auditory memory (Church and Abel, 1998). Auditory memory is the ability to store speech stimuli. Auditory memory is closely related to auditory sequencing and discrimination abilities (Reed, 1994). Auditory memory is also in close relationship to processing skills. In order for auditory stimuli to be differentiated, the speech signal must be remembered long enough to be compared. If this does not happen, processing cannot completely take place and the message has not been carried through.

Cognitive abilities and language skills can be negatively affected by problems with attention. Attention to various environmental stimuli is a necessary prerequisite for the acquisition of concepts that underlie language. Likewise, it is imperative to only attenuate to certain stimuli in the environment and ignore extraneous stimuli so that the intended message can be grasped.

Even the Native American FAS children who exhibited no signs of mental retardation or any dysmorphic features still had communication impairments. Eighty percent of Native American children with FAS over the age of one year demonstrate "impairments in speech and language acquisition, voice and fluency, the basis for which could not be associated with hearing defects" (Reed, 1994).

Native American children with FAS develop language at a much lower rate than younger normal children of similar linguistic age (Becker, Warr-Leeper, and Leeper, 1990). When compared to normal children of the same linguistic age, the FAS children were also unable to produce grammatical sentences with the same degree of syntactic complexity. They could, however, understand and comprehend grammatical forms at similar levels.

Pragmatically, North American Indian children with FAS understand turn taking in conversation, but they had problems deciphering the pragmatic intent of the previous statement. Therefore, their responses were pragmatically inappropriate (Becker, Warr-Leeper, and Leeper, 1990). In this regard, they can be likened unto the SLI child. FAS children appear to lack the conversational postulate necessary for communication effectiveness. They lack the ability to show reference. Becker, Warr-Leeper, and Leeper (1990) also proved that FAS children are more likely to produce grammatically inaccurate and incomplete sentences in spontaneous conversation than the younger normal children are. For instance, the adult caretaker asks the child, *did you color in your coloring book at school today?* The child responds, *I had to sit in my desk.* Obviously, the adult feels that this response is inappropriate and attempts to make the response meaningful, saying . . . *you had to sit in your desk to color today.* In actuality that was not the case. The child was not allowed to color because he had been disruptive and was forced to sit in his desk for a "time-out" during coloring time. It is necessary to probe the FAS child so that the message can be accurately decoded.

These children also exhibit a much higher rate of articulation impairments in comparison to normal children. FAS children tend to have much more nasal or velar assimilation. FAS children also tend to make odd substitutions. For instance, one five-year-old boy kept using /g/ in substitution for /t s/ and /s/ in the initial position of words. He also demonstrated lateral air emission on final /s/; gliding of liquids /j/, /r/ and final /l/; fronting of palatal alveolars /s/, /z/ and final /s/; and cluster reduction of /s/ clusters (Becker, Warr-Leeper, and Leeper, 1990).

Morphologically and syntactically, the FAS children did not demonstrate comprehension for picture identification to the same degree as the younger control group. Like SLI children, FAS children also show deficits in the ability to successfully store and retrieve language examples as needed (Becker Warr-Leeper, and Leeper, 1990).

However, one cannot forget that the majority of Native North American children are affected at least in some degree to bilingualism. As of yet there has been no research conducted on the effects of bilingualism on children with FAS. However, normal bilingual children experience brief periods in language acquisition when they are not developing at the same rate as monolingual children. Normal developing bilingual children catch up with monolingual children. Also, children affected by bilingualism tend to have articulation difficulties. It would be interesting to study whether the effects of bilingualism could be an attributing factor to the disproportionate amount of problems seen in Native Americans with FAS.

FAS is devastating Native American communities. FAS and FAE are diseases that give birth to an overwhelming amount of communication problems. Hearing losses and language disorders are prevalent among this special population of individuals. Native Americans throughout history have shown a cultural weakness to the effects of alcohol. This predisposed genetic weakness is only confounded upon when poverty, lack of education, and perhaps even bilingualism are added to the mix. It is becoming necessary that SLPs learn to recognize the symptoms of FAS and FAE and learn how to work with the special individuals who suffer from these disorders.

FAS AMONG AFRICAN AMERICANS

Brianna is a nine-year-old African-American girl who is currently a fourth grade student. Although she interacts well with the other children, she is noticeably smaller in stature compared to the rest of her class. Brianna is only forty-five inches tall and weighs thirty-eight pounds. She is being raised in a single parent home by her father. She also suffers from several other disorders, which include cleft lip and palate, moderate hearing loss, poor visual acuity, and hand tremors. Academically, Brianna struggles on a day-to-day basis to keep up with her class. Overall, Brianna's language skills are considered to be below average for her age. Despite her numerous disabilities, Brianna maintains a pleasant disposition. It is apparent that Brianna's numerous health problems contribute to her academic difficulties. Brianna's mother admitted that she consumed alcohol excessively during her pregnancy with Brianna. This behavior made her defenseless unborn baby girl Brianna a victim of FAS.

Like Brianna's mother, the number of African-American women who consume alcohol during pregnancy is higher than that of white women (National Clearinghouse for Alcohol and Drug Information, 1998). Therefore, the number of children with FAS is also high. In order to better understand the effects of FAS on African Americans, we must first examine the patterns of alcohol use and abuse in addition to some of the contributing factors among the culture.

If we reflect on the history of African Americans in the United States, we are all aware of the dismal beginnings for this race of people. They were separated from their homeland and families and forced into a life of servitude. African Americans were stripped of every shred of dignity and told they were less than human and deserved no rights or freedoms in the United States. Although slavery ended, racism managed to persist. African Americans had to struggle for the same liberties and justices as whites. For many Americans, alcohol was a means of escaping the stress and tension that existed in a cold, bitter, segregated society. Naturally, children emulate what they see and adapt the habits and behaviors of their environment. In many ways the use of alcohol in the African-American community is a carryover from earlier generations. Today, there is a significant amount of successful African Americans who have not fallen prey to the demons of alcohol, but there are still a considerable number of African Americans who live in low socioeconomic environments and continue to consume alcohol as a means of escaping their problems.

Alcoholism crosses all racial boundaries. However, there does not seem to be any single factor, which contributes to the high incidence of alcoholism among African Americans. Researchers seem to indicate that there may be several contributing factors, which include socioeconomic status, cultural influence, geographic location, nutrition, and metabolic differences. Sources indicate that the lifetime prevalence of alcoholism is higher for African-American men and women between thirty and sixty years of age, while between the ages of eighteen and twenty-nine and following age sixty, the prevalence of alcohol use is lower for African Americans (National Clearinghouse for Alcohol and Drug Information, 1998). It seems as though younger African Americans are less likely to use alcohol than whites of the same age. Even though lifetime prevalence is somewhat higher in African Americans, there is little difference between African Americans and whites in the lifetime prevalence of alcoholism (National Center for Environmental Health, 1998). In general, deaths occurring from alcohol-induced cause (liver disease, malignancy of digestive organs, vehicular accidents, or homicide) are approximately two-and-a-half times greater within the African-American population, compared to that of whites.

When examining specific patterns of alcohol use among women, there are some additional factors that need to be considered. These factors include age, education, and marital status. Data gathered by the U.S. Department of Health and Human Resources (1990) indicate that between African-American and white women, we see that there are higher numbers of abstainers (women who consume zero drinks) among younger African-American women and women over sixty. On the other hand, there was a higher incidence of heavy drinkers (those who consume one or more ounces of alcohol per day) among middle-aged African-American women, although African-American women tend to drink less on the average than white women.

SUMMARY

FAS is classified as an alcohol-related birth defect, which describes a range of anatomic or functional abnormalities. Generally, birth defects attributed to FAS can include prenatal or postnatal growth retardation as well as CNS deficits. These deficits would include neurological abnormalities, developmental delays, behavioral malformations, intellectual impairment, and skull or brain malformations. Malformations obviously affect the general appearance of the child. Typical characteristics of the face include short eye openings, a very thin upper lip, and the mid-face and philtrum are elongated and flattened. Cleft lip and palate are also attributed to alcohol consumption during pregnancy. Mental handicaps and hyperactivity are also among the most common and debilitating aspects of FAS. "Deficits in learning ability, attention and memory and problem solving are prevalent, in addition to fine and gross motor skills, impulsiveness and speech and hearing impairments" (Sparks, 1993). The deficits that many of these children face during their early lives carries over into adolescence and adulthood.

While FAS is a viable disorder, there is no actual test that can be administered to determine whether a child is suffering from this disorder. FAS is generally diagnosed based upon clinical judgment and manifestation of deficiencies observed in the child. The term FAE is frequently used as well. FAE is considered to be a less severe set of the same symptoms of FAS. One thing that is not clearly understood is whether or not "FAS and FAE are two distinctive disorders, or if they are merely extremes of a continuum of a single condition: Alcohol related Birth Defects" (Sparks, 1993).

As a child grows from infancy to adulthood there are many milestones that are achieved along the way particularly, in language development. If we consider the factors attributed to FAS, then we can recognize how low socioeconomic status and cultural difference can hinder the language development of a normally developing child. Therefore, the FAS child is at an even greater risk for having language delays. If alcohol continues to be a factor in the home environment, then the child may have limited verbal stimulation and minimal interactions with peers or adults. In addition, motor skills may be delayed, thereby thwarting the child's ability to wander around and explore the environment and develop that "internal" language that Piaget speaks about so often.

When the FAS child approaches the school-age years, language deficit become more apparent because expectations are higher. "Some typical language problems that are evident include: verbal comprehension, reading comprehension, receptive and expressive vocabulary, long and short term memory, short attention span and socialization skills" (Sparks, 1993). Many times these children become frustrated in school and can become behavior problems for teachers. As the child progresses toward adolescence, behavior in school continues to be an issue and there is a greater tendency for the FAS child to either be suspended, expelled, or to drop out of school. Some of the reasons for this include difficulty in getting along with other children, disobedience or disrespect toward teachers and truancy (National Center for Environmental Health, 1998). Adolescence is a difficult growth and adjustment period for the typical child, but for an FAS child these times are even more volatile. Once FAS children reach adulthood they "generally have difficulty sustaining employment or living independently as productive members of their community" (U.S. Department of Health and Human Services, 1998).

REFERENCES

Abkarian, C.G. (1992). Communication Effects of Prenatal Alcohol Exposure. *Journal of Communication Disorders.* 25, 221-240.

Bach, M., and L. Wasson (1991). Fetal Alcohol Syndrome. *Advance.* 3(3), 25-28.

Becker, M., G.A. Warr-Leeper, and H.A. Leeper. Fetal Alcohol Syndrome: A Description of Oral Motor, Articulatory, Short Term Memory, Grammatical, and Semantic Abilities. *Journal of Communication Disorders.* April 1990; 23(2), 97-124.

Carney, L.J., and G.D. Chermak. Performance of American Indian Children with Fetal Alcohol Syndrome on the Test of Language Development. *Journal of Communication Disorders.* April 1991, 24(2), 123-134.

Church, M.W. and E.L. Abel. Fetal Alcohol Syndrome. Hearing, Speech, Language, and Vestibular Disorders. *Obstetrics and Gynecological Clinical Journal of North America.* March 1998, 25(1), 85-97.

Day, N.L. (1992). The Effects of Prenatal Exposure to Alcohol. *Alcohol Health & Research World.* 16(3), 238-243.

Gale, T.C., White, J.A., and T.K. Welty. Difference in Detection of Alcohol Use in a Prenatal Population (on a Northern Plains Indian Reservation) Using Various Methods of Ascertainment. *S.D.J. Med.* July 1998, 51(7), 235-240.

Hamilton, M.A. (1981). Linguistic Abilities of Children with Fetal Alcohol Syndrome. Ann Arbor, MI: University Microfilms International.

Jones, K. and D. Smith (1973). Recognition of the Fetal Alcohol Syndrome in Early Infancy. *Lancet.* 999-1001.

Kellerman, Teresa. Who is at Risk of FAS/FAE. Available at: http://www.fas.htm.

Kinsley, M. (May 17, 1991). Drinking for Two. *The Washington Post,* A25.

Larroque, B., Kaminski, M., Dechaene, P., Subtil, D., Delfosse, M., and D. Querleu (1995). Moderate Prenatal Alcohol Exposure and Psychomotor Development at Preschool Age. *American Journal of Public Health.* 85, 1654-1661.

Lemonine, P., Harrousseau, H., Borteyru, J.P., and J.C. Menuet (1968). Les Enfants De Parents Alcooloques: Anomalies Obsevees a Propos de 127 Cas. *Quest Medical.* 21, 476-482.

Ma, G.X., Toubbeh, J., Cline, J., and A. Chisholm. Native American Adolescents' Views of Fetal Alcohol Syndrome Prevention in School. *Journal of School Health.* April 1998; 68(4), 131-136.

National Center for Environmental Health. Secondary Conditions of Fetal Alcohol Syndrome (1998). Washington, DC: Author.

National Clearinghouse for Alcohol and Drug Information. Alcohol, Tobacco and other Drugs and Pregnancy and Parenthood (1998). New York: Author.

National Institute on Alcohol Abuse and Alcoholism. *Alcohol Alert.* No. 13 PH 297 July 1991.

The National Organization on Fetal Alcohol Syndrome. Fetal Alcohol Syndrome (1998). Washington, DC: Author.

Native American Women's Health Education Resource Center. Available at: http://www.occee.ou.edu/aii/fas.html.

Reed, V.V. (1994). *An Introduction to Children with Language Disorder.* Second Edition. New York: McMillan Coll. Pub. 157, 163, 41, 44.

7th Generation Project. Available at: http://www/occe.ou.edu/aii/fas.html.

Sparks, Shirley N. (1993). *Children of Prenatal Substance Abuse.* San Diego, CA: Singular Publishing Group, Inc.

Streissguth, Ann. (1997). *Fetal Alcohol Syndrome: A Guide for Families and Communities.* Paul H. Brookes Publishing Co. 9-35.

U.S. Department of Health and Human Services. (1990). *Alcohol, Tobacco, and Other Drugs May Harm the Unborn.* (ADM) 90-1711. Washington, DC: Author.

U.S. Department of Health and Human Services. Fetal Alcohol Syndrome Prevention (1998). Washington, DC: Author.

Vobejda, B. (April 20, 1994). Sobering Look at Alcohol and Pregnancy; Doctors Face the Facts on Drinking's Effects. *The Washington Post,* Ae.

Chapter 9

Treatment and Family Counseling of Drug-Exposed Children

PREGNANCY AND DRUG-USE TRENDS

Approximately half of the women who abuse illegal drugs are within the childbearing age group of fifteen to forty-four years of age. In 1992 and 1993, the National Institute on Drug Abuse (NIDA), a division of the National Institute of Health, conducted a national hospital survey to determine the extent of drug abuse among pregnant women in the United States. It was called the National Pregnancy and Health survey, and it currently serves as the most recent national data available (National Institute on Drug Abuse, 1994).

This survey revealed that of the 4 million women who gave birth during the survey period, 757,000 drank alcohol and smoked cigarettes during their pregnancies. There was an association between cigarette, alcohol, and illegal drug usage. Thirty-two percent of the women who mentioned using one drug also smoked cigarettes and drank alcohol (National Institute on Drug Abuse, 1994).

The results of the survey showed that 221,000 women used illegal drugs during their pregnancies, with marijuana and cocaine being the most common drugs used. The number of women who used marijuana was 119,000 in comparison to the 45,000 who reported the use of cocaine. The rates of illegal drugs usage was higher in women who were single, had less than sixteen years of formal education, were not employed, and relied on some source of funding to pay for their hospital stay.

HIV, Substance Abuse, and Communication Disorders in Children
© 2007 by The Haworth Press, Inc. All rights reserved.
doi:10.1300/5438_09

Most of the women who abuse drugs do so from three months before pregnancy to the conclusion of the pregnancy. Another NIDA study indicated that women who are successfully detoxified and enrolled in treatment programs are motivated to remain drug-free in order to care for their children.

COMMON DRUGS OF ABUSE
AND THEIR EFFECTS ON BABIES

Following is a list of substances and their effects on infants who have been prenatally exposed to other substances.

1. Babies who have had prenatal exposure to alcohol have an abnormally low birth weight and are shorter in length. They also may have a small head circumference, facial deformities, and FAS.
2. Infants who have been exposed to tobacco products have a low birth weight, frequently have premature births, and are at increased risk of Sudden Infant Death Syndrome or SIDS.
3. Prenatal marijuana exposure may result in a premature birth, low birth weight, body tremors, and irritability.
4. Cocaine-exposed infants display increased crying, low birth weight, a short body length, difficulty eating or sleeping, and vomiting between feedings.
5. Prenatal crack exposure results in a small head circumference, low birth weight, premature birth, increased crying, difficulty in eating or sleeping, increased irritability, and inconsolable behavior.
6. Infants who are prenatally exposed to heroin display a low birth weight, increased crying, and difficulty in eating or sleeping.
7. Finally, PCP or LSD exposure is demonstrated through behavior difficulties and violent temper tantrums.

IDENTIFYING NEONATE ADDICTION

"Crack babies" are frequently born prematurely with a low gestational birth weight. Within twenty-four hours of birth, these infants will exhibit the onset of tremors, hyperactive reflexes, irritability, increased muscle tone, twitching, increased mucous production, nasal congestion, respiratory distress, excessive sweating, increase in temperature, vomiting, diarrhea, and dehydration. The symptoms displayed by crack babies must be separated from the symptoms of other illnesses before a diagnosis can be made.

Crack babies have shrill cries, sneeze frequently due to nasal congestion, frantically suck their fists but do not eat well, and may yawn although they have difficulty falling asleep. They are unusually pale, are candidates for seizures, and are often born with nose and knee abrasions; however, the presence of the abrasions is not understood.

The symptoms seen in crack babies may be caused by several drugs other than crack, and include heroin, methadone, diazepam, phenobarbital, and alcohol.

Unique Aspects of Drug-Exposed Infants

Drug-exposed infants are usually from the poorest populations of society. In addition to the problems of nutrition and health, children raised in poverty are likely to face homelessness, violence, and crime. Poverty is also associated with minority status, race, and ethnicity. Cultural factors may affect the use of drugs and childbearing practices.

Teenage mothers comprise a group that places infants into double jeopardy. Initially, teenage motherhood is viewed as a prenatal risk situation due to the fact that teenage mothers may not have the adequate financial resources to care for their children. It is believed that some teenage mothers are not able to provide sufficient parental support due to their lack of emotional development.

Social service agencies are usually involved with drug-exposed infants since these children are, in many cases, targets of child abuse and neglect. Some children may encounter several caretakers and as many as eight foster care placements in their first year of life (Beckwith et al.,1994).

EFFECTS OF COCAINE USE

Cocaine use during pregnancy may affect neuroregulatory mechanisms that result in behavior regulation.

Standardized Testing of Cocaine-Exposed Preschool and School-Age Children

In earlier reports of cocaine exposure, the exposure was thought to be linked to moderate to severe developmental delays across all domains. More recent studies have shown mild to no impairments in the overall developmental functioning in cocaine-exposed children (Chasnoff, Landress, and Barrett, 1990). The developmental profiles of a group of 106 cocaine/alcohol-exposed twenty-four-month-olds followed from birth were compared with performance of forty-five toddlers exposed to marijuana and/or alcohol but not cocaine and seventy-seven nondrug-exposed children. The mothers of infants in the two comparison groups were similar to the cocaine-using mothers in socioeconomic status, age, marital status, and tobacco use during pregnancy. On repeated developmental assessments using the Bayley Scales at three, six, twelve, eighteen, and twenty-four months, there were no significant differences in either the mental or motor domains, although the investigators mentioned that a higher percentage of cocaine-exposed infants scored two standard deviations below the mean (Chasnoff et al., 1990). The cocaine-exposed children from this group showed no differences on overall performance on the Stanford-Binet Intelligence Scale from the noncocaine-exposed controls (Griffith, Azuma, and Chasnoff, 1994). The cocaine-exposed group scored significantly lower on verbal reasoning tasks.

Language and Symbolic Play

Language development and the capacity for symbolic play are closely related since both involve maturing capacities for representation and communication. Play in the first year of life is mainly nonsymbolic, but play in the second and third years involves the capacity for substituting function, such as using a cup to represent an object other than a cup, and for pretending. The movement from nonsymbolic to symbolic play occurs gradually. There are individual differences in the range of symbolic play shown by children in their second year of life. At thirteen months, some toddlers engage in symbolic play shown by children in their second year of life. At thirteen months, some toddlers engage in symbolic play (Tamis-LeMonda and Bornstein, 1990, 1991). The capacity for symbolic play at thirteen months may be used to predict a child's development at twenty months of age and older.

There are several sources of individual variation in the development of abilities for language and play, including differences in overall cognitive competency, but there are two sources that relate to areas of concern for children prenatally exposed to cocaine. Firstly, language development depends upon a child's ability to maintain attention and to explore his or her environment. Problems in arousal and alertness will indirectly affect the emergence of language. Secondly, maternal stimulation increases children's use of language and level of symbolic and nonsymbolic play (Tamis-LeMonda and Bornstein, 1990, 1991). A combination of maternal social (e.g., physical, affectionate contact) and attention directing (or didactic) activities affect a toddler's complexity of play. Mothers who abuse cocaine may be more likely to have difficulty with the kinds of interactive tasks that support both language and play development. Drug-exposed children are less likely to engage in symbolic play or nonsymbolic exploration and exhibit disorganized, poorly modulated play such as scattering and throwing toys (Rodning, Beckwith, and Howard, 1989).

SPEECH AND LANGUAGE INTERVENTION

The manner in which services are delivered may vary from child to child since there are various methods of intervention. Parents and caregivers play a large role in the early language learning of toddlers and preschoolers. A common recommendation for children with language impairments is placement in a preschool program (Reed, 1994).

A frequently used strategy involves training the child's parents or caregivers. This method focuses on (1) creating or enhancing the child's environment to facilitate change in the child's language, and (2) responding within that environment in a manner that best facilitates language change.

At least two primary aspects are involved in changing or enhancing the child's language-learning environment. One method focuses on helping the parents or caregivers recognize and take advantage of language-learning opportunities that occur in the child's daily activities. This approach stresses seizing opportunities and capitalizing on language-teaching moments. These moments may include dressing, interactive play, meal or snack time, story time, or any other time during the day when the child's attention is centered on a specific action, object, or event. The parents and caregivers are shown how to identify these events and how to structure their language and gestures accordingly. The second method involves creating opportunities for language learning. The parents and caregivers are shown how to set up moments in the environment to encourage the child's use of specific language behaviors during those periods (Reed, 1994).

The goal in involving parents and caregivers is to show them which of their behaviors should be increased or decreased. An example of changes in parental language would be a reduction in the frequency of directive speech acts, including commands and demands for responses from the children, and an increase in their use of (1) responsive speech acts, (2) information-seeking questions when the information presumably is not known to the adult, (3) confirmation requests to affirm that the adult understood the child correctly, and (4) simple repetitions of the child's utterances to maintain their content, but in a form that slightly modifies the one used by the child (Reed, 1994).

Treatment for the behaviors of the drug-exposed child includes medication and counseling the parents. Research has shown that early intervention, appropriate for high-risk children, also benefits the drug-exposed child (Sparks, 1993). Although intervention and treatment of this population remains an arena that could benefit from more research, several studies have provided valuable information pertaining to treatment. Intervention for the drug-exposed child greatly depends on the substance that the mother abused while pregnant. Recent research provides intervention for cocaine, opium, and amphetamine exposure. However, research has shown that some general techniques can be utilized when the exact drug is known. Some of these are now discussed.

Cocaine

The cocaine-exposed child may need behavior treatment, which may involve therapies and techniques to alleviate irritability, passiveness, or frantic crying. However, research has also shown that most children exposed to cocaine prenatally are unaffected (Sparks, 1993). We can imply from these conclusions that the range of behaviors exhibited by infants and toddlers of this population are indeed vast, which encourages the implementation of an individualized program of structured interactions. Longitudinal studies conducted by the National Association for Perinatal Addiction Research and Education (NAPARE) and the Los Angeles Unified School District's Prenatally Exposed to Drugs (PED) Programs have provided information regarding intervention of this population (Sparks, 1993). They have developed several procedures that should be followed by caregivers, teachers, and service workers involved in the treatment of drug-exposed children.

The caregiver must carefully observe for signs of distress exhibited by the infant. These signs include yawns, sneezes, increased muscle tone and flailing, irritability, disorganized sucking, and crying. Sparks (1993) believes that when these signs are noticed, the caregiver must allow time for the infant to "recover control" and then return to the interaction in his/her own time. An individualized program of structured physical contact is appropriate.

Massaging the cocaine-exposed infant has been found to be beneficial. Infants who had been massaged for thirty minutes per day for ten days gained more weight, were less irritable, showed superior habituation scores, exhibited higher vagal tone, and had significantly higher norepinephrine and dopamine levels (Fields and Scafidi, 1998).

Controlling the environments of the infant is essential to prevent overstimulation. Drastic changes should not be present in the child's environment. Stimulation should be introduced to the infant one dimension at a time. Sparks (1993) suggests voice-only stimulation or face only, preceding both voice and face stimulation. During interaction, caregivers should use soft voices and make adequate eye contact (Chiang and Finnegan, 1995). Alterations to the room, such as using smaller, clearly defined spaces with low shelves, screens, and furniture are considerations (Sparks, 1993).

The cocaine-exposed infant requires little pharmacotherapy. Phenobarbital can be administered the first few days after birth if signs of irritability are noted. This drug also controls seizures as a result of the cocaine exposure (Chiang and Finnegan, 1995).

Opium

When the infant has been exposed to opium in utero, it is beneficial also to handle the child gently, based on the infant's body language and other cues. According to a study conducted by Oro and Dixon, placement on a nonoscillating waterbed has been found to benefit this child (Chiang and Finnegan, 1995). Infants who were exposed to this waterbed and medication therapy had better weight gain than those infants who were treated with pharmacotherapy alone.

Pharmocotherapy has been found effective in treating the absti-nence symptoms that many of these infants and children exhibit. If these symptoms are not treated, the infant may die from excessive fluid loss, respiratory distress, seizures, vomiting and aspiration, or hyper-pyrexia (Chiang and Finnegan,1995). Naloxone is a drug that is used to contraindicate the effects of opium on the exposed infant. It is often first given to the exposed newborn in the delivery room. Frequently, a substitute opium or a nonspecific CNS depressant is used in treatment.

Environment conditions, such as dim lighting, soft bedding, and swaddling in a side-lying position have also a benefit to the opium-exposed child. Supplying the infant with adequate fluids and calories is another supportive treatment measure which aids the infant in maintaining the appropriate weight (Chiang and Finnegan, 1995).

Amphetamines

The impact of amphetamines is similar to those of cocaine. Several studies conducted in Sweden by Erikson and colleagues found many of these identical symptoms. However, the treatment of the amphet-amine-exposed newborn was not reported (Chiang and Finnegan, 1995).

Intervention for the drug-exposed child should involve the primary caregiver so that there will be consistency in treatment in all environ-ments. Parents benefit significantly from inclusion in the assessment and the treatment of their infants. Both the mother and the father of the infant should be included (Chiang and Finnegan, 1995). If the child is preschool or school-aged, an Individual Family Service Plan (IFSP) is necessary for maximal family involvement (Sparks, 1993). In addition, other goals should be developed with the caregiver. The primary goal of intervention for the mother is to improve her feelings of competence as a parent. Goals of recovery for her and parental goals should be carefully balanced to promote success (Sparks, 1993).

Current research provides professionals with some insight and suggestions for intervening with this challenging population. However, more research is needed to adequately answer questions regarding treatment of the drug-exposed child.

REFERENCES

Beckwith, L., Rodning, C., Norris, D., Phillipsen, L., Khandabi, P., and J. Howard (1994). Spontaneous Play in Two-Year-Olds Born to Substance Abusing Mothers. *Infant Mental Health Journal.* 15(2), 128-135.

Chasnoff, I.J., Landress, H., and M. Barrett (1990). The Prevalence of Illicit Drug or Alcohol Use During Pregnancy and Discrepancies in Reporting in Pinellas County, Florida. *New England Journal of Medicine.* 322, 1202-1206.

Chiang, C. and Finnegan, L., National Institute on Drug Abuse (1995). *Medications Development for the Treatment of Pregnant Addicts and Their Infants* (NIDA Research Monograph, 149). Washington, DC: U.S. Department of Health and Human Services.

Fields, T. and F. Scafidi (1998). Polydrug-Using Adolescent Mothers and Their Infants Receiving Early Intervention. *Adolescence.* 33(129), 177-144.

Griffith, D.R., Azuma, S.D., and I.J.Chasnoff (1994). Three-Year Outcome of Children Exposed Prenatally to Drugs. *Journal of the American Academy of Child Psychiatry.* 33, 20-27.

National Institute on Drug Abuse (1994).

Reed, V.A. (1994). *An Introduction to Children with Language Disorders,* Second Edition. New York: Maxwell Macmillan International. 144.

Rodning, C., Beckwith, L., and J. Howard (1989). Characteristics of Attachment Organization and Play Organization in Prenatally Drug-Exposed Toddlers. *Developmental Psychopathology.* 1, 277-289.

Sparks, S. (1993). *Children of Prenatal Substance Abuse.* San Diego, CA: Singular Publishing.

Tamis-LeMonda, C.S. and M.H. Bornstein (1990). Language, Play, and Attention at One Year. *Infant Behavior Development.* 13, 85-89.

———. (1991). Individual Variation Correspondence, Stability, and Change in Mother and Toddler Play. *Infant Behavior Development.* 14, 143-162.

Chapter 10

Case Studies

Clinicians will find information about the typical experiences of children with a history of substance abuse and/or HIV useful. Clinicians who know typical and atypical patterns of behaviors can develop evidenced-based clinical intervention plans. A great deal of information exists about the physical, medical, and cognitive factors that distinguish children with a history of substance abuse and/or HIV from normally developing children and from other communicatively disordered children. Such clinical evidence provides clinicians with a foundation for selecting assessment protocols, interpreting results, and developing intervention goals. The evidence also provides a basis for distinguishing behavioral differences from communication disorders.

The information clinicians need about family patterns of children from this population is less available. Information about family structure and dynamics provides clinicians with a framework for selecting appropriate service delivery methods. It may be that some communicatively disordered children with a history of substance abuse and/or HIV will benefit from traditional home-based intervention plans. Others may require participation of persons generally not thought to serve primary roles in such intervention plans. Still others may require interventions to occur in settings not previously considered.

In this final chapter, we present a series of case studies illustrating the communication disorders of this special population. Children who have experienced prenatal exposure to substance abuse and/or HIV frequently belong to families in trouble. To address the needs of com-

HIV, Substance Abuse, and Communication Disorders in Children
© 2007 by The Haworth Press, Inc. All rights reserved.
doi:10.1300/5438_10

municatively disordered children from this population, a clinician will need information about the ways substance abuse and HIV alter family dynamics and the roles played by family members in a child's development under these circumstances. This chapter provides some information about the family structures and dynamics observed in four cases.

CASE ONE

Cindy was born at thirty-six weeks gestation with a birth weight of four pounds, ten ounces, a diagnosis of small for gestational age (SGA), jaundice, and a positive toxicology screen for methamphetamines. She has a diagnosis of FAS, Type 3. The diagnosis is based on a well-documented history of drug and alcohol exposure, birth weight, parameters for length, weight, and head circumference, increased muscle tone, mid-face hypoplasia, remarkable appearance of the philtrum, and a high-arched palate. Cindy spent the first nine days of life in the NICU to gain weight.

Ms. Wright is Cindy's twenty-four-year-old biological mother. Ms. Wright is Caucasian with a Polish, Italian, and Catholic background. She completed high school and currently works as a cashier in a local grocery store. She attended rehabilitation for substance abuse and alcoholism on three separate occasions beginning at the age of sixteen. She is currently sober and attends AA meetings on a regular basis. Cindy's father is, according to Ms. Wright, an automotive mechanic that she met at the age of nineteen. He is Hispanic, but Ms. Wright has never met his family and does not know much about them.

According to Ms. Wright, Cindy spent her first nine days of life in the NICU to gain weight. Upon release from the NICU, Cindy went home to live with her mother and maternal grandmother. Cindy's father now lives in another state with Cindy's four-year-old half-sister. Cindy's maternal grandfather passed away five years earlier from liver failure related to alcoholism. Cindy and her mother stayed with the grandmother until Cindy was about one year of age. At that time, Ms. Wright, (Cindy's mother) felt financially secure enough to live on her own supporting Cindy and herself. Cindy now lives with her mother and mother's boyfriend.

Cindy lives in a midsized urban city on the East coast. She lives in an apartment building, nine stories high, with ten apartments on each floor. There are laundry facilities in the basement and playground behind the building. The lawn around the building is well groomed and there is a flower garden in front. The residents are a diverse group, with whites, blacks, and Hispanics, mostly young, single, or single with children. In Cindy's block, there are four apartment buildings, a gas station, a liquor store, a grocery store, and a dry cleaner.

Cindy continues to receive home visits from Social Services because of her diagnosis of FAS. While her mother works, Cindy stays with her grandmother two days out of the week (the grandmother's days off), her mother's boyfriend, two days out of the week (his days off), and with a neighbor who keeps four other children, on Fridays. This arrangement allows Cindy's mother to pay for only one day a week of childcare.

Based on the Denver Developmental Screening II, Cindy's personal–social skills were determined to be within normal limits, fine motor and gross motor skills were within normal limits, but that there were delays present in the area of expressive language skills.

Based on this information, Cindy was scheduled for a return visit two weeks later. On the second visit, the Early Learning Accomplishment Profile was administered. At nineteen months of age, Cindy's gross motor skills were found to be age appropriate. Her fine motor skills were found to be at sixteen months, and cognitive skills were found to be at eighteen months. Self-help skills were found to be at eighteen months, social/emotional skills were found to be at seventeen months, and language skills were found to be at fifteen months. She followed simple directions, without cues, retrieved named objects, and recognized a picture of a ball. She attended well to pictures in a book and demonstrated a good attention span for her age. She demonstrated understanding verbs in context such as "give bear something to eat." She did not demonstrate understanding of pronouns such as "my, your" or spatial concepts such as "in, on, off." She did not readily initiate words during the evaluation, and said only a few spontaneous words. Once rapport was established with the examiner, Cindy started initiating interactions such as handing the examiner toys to show them to her. She vocalized "W" to name/comment on what she saw as she looked out of the window and said "dada" while handing her father the bubbles to communicate that she wanted him to open them. During a repetitive game of blowing bubbles, she said "ba" for "bubbles" consistently and "baba" for "bubbles" one time to request more bubbles. She was not yet able to blow bubbles. She consistently said "more" spontaneously to request more of an activity given a pause or delay in routine. She also vocalized a sound (meow) for cat when she saw a picture of cat and imitated a car motor and airplane sounds. She named only one object on request ("ba" for "ball") during the evaluation. During child-directed play, Cindy jargoned with strings of syllables such as "horti-dana."

During play in the room with three other children and one adult, Cindy was observed to take a ball from the toy box and hold it. After a few minutes, the adult engaged Cindy in ball rolling and she readily engaged. She also readily accepted the other children joining in the game. After approximately eight minutes, Cindy left the game to look at a book. When the adult joined her for book reading, she pointed to pictures when named. Cindy played peek-a-boo with the other children upon their nonverbal request and soon they began to eagerly chase one another around the room.

Ms. Wright (mother) stated that Cindy is able to identify her body parts and that she primarily points and gestures to communicate at home. Ms.

Wright also reported that Cindy is able to say thirty words (including pee-pee, mama, dada, grandma). She reportedly will look for named items that are not in sight at home (such as go get your diaper). At the end of the language evaluation, the audiologist conducted the hearing evaluation. Responses to pure tones were within normal limits bilaterally. Speech awareness levels were in agreement with pure tone findings. Tympanometry was within normal limits bilaterally.

A third appointment diagnostic findings were reviewed and treatment planning begun. This nearly twenty-month-old toddler is at a language-age equivalency range of fifteen to eighteen months, indicating that she is mildly delayed. During this session, the clinician modeled three language stimulation techniques for Ms. Wright, her boyfriend, and grandmother to use when playing with Cindy. Cindy was observed to be very responsive to the language stimulation techniques. The techniques included modeling the labels for people, objects, and actions, expanding the Cindy's utterances to add a name or action depending on context and prompting Cindy to count objects "1,2,3" and to say "please and thank you." An additional component of the plan was to encourage routine mealtimes to increase weight gain. Given this goal, Cindy's caretakers were encouraged to not engage in language stimulation activities at that time. Nutritionists were to monitor weight gain.

Questions

- How would you validate the data concerning Cindy's physical, medical, and social history?
- Is the treatment plan appropriate? Which aspects of the plan led you to make your conclusion?
- What additional questions might be asked to learn about family and daily routines? How would you incorporate the additional information into the treatment plan?

CASE TWO

Eric is a fourteen-month-old male infant referred for evaluation because of in-utero drug exposure. His father is twenty-five years old and has been convicted of child abuse and neglect. His mother is nineteen years old and has a reported history of substance abuse. Currently, Eric is in the care of a foster family and has been since the age of three months.

At birth, Eric had a positive toxicology screen for cocaine, codeine, and morphine. Child Protective Services removed him from his home, at three months of age, because of reports of abuse and because he appeared malnourished and underweight. Medical examination revealed that at three months of age, Eric weighed six pounds and twelve ounces. Upon examination, he demonstrated head lag when pulled up, was startled at light and sound, but smiled appropriately. His height was in the 25th percentile, his weight was in the 50th percentile, and head circumference was in the 75th percentile.

Speech and language skills were age appropriate at seven months, but left tympanogram revealed negative pressure with poor eardrum mobility (middle-ear fluid). Right tympanogram revealed negative pressure with good eardrum movement. Otocaoustic emissions were present bilaterally. A startle was elicited in sound field at 80dB. Response to pure tones and speech awareness level was within normal limits for right ear but not for left ear.

At fourteen months, left tympanogram revealed negative pressure with poor eardrum mobility. Right tympanogram revealed negative pressure with good ear mobility. A binaural speech awareness level was obtained within normal limits. Language skills were assessed using the Rosetti Infant-Toddler Language Scale and the Infant Scale of Communicative Intent. These developmental checklists determined that Eric was functioning at the eleven to twelve month level for receptive and expressive language skills. An eligibility meeting determined that eligibility for special services would be deferred and that a reevaluation be scheduled around Eric's second birthday. Moreover, Eric would be going for visits with his biological mother beginning in three weeks to help determine the possibility of them being reunited.

Questions

- How would you plan to help Eric's caregivers keep track of his developmental milestones, keeping in mind his current and future living arrangements?
- How would you assist Eric's caregivers in team building to best meet Eric's developmental needs?
- What recommendations do you suspect the audiologist may make on Eric's behalf?

CASE THREE

Seventeen-month-old Mary Anne was brought in for assessment with concerns of developmental delay thought to be associated with drug exposure in utero, microcephaly, and possible FAS. Her biological parents are in their thirties and unemployed. They are both drug and alcohol abusers. It was reported that Mary Anne's mother had no prenatal care. Mary Anne was born at thirty-two weeks gestation with a birth weight of five pounds and one ounce. The baby had a positive toxicology screen (amphetamines and alcohol). The child was LGA (large for gestational age) related to maternal gestational diabetes. The child was hospitalized for one month at the age of six months for reflux surgery and for one week for RSV at the age of one year. The child has a history of respiratory distress, left-sided pneumothorax, apnea, gastroesophageal reflux and fundoplication, RSV, laryngeal malacia, and cyanotic breath holding spells. The child has had three cases of otitis media within the past five months. She has a history of seizure with fever and roseola. The child has been in her present foster home since five months of age.

Her foster mother reported that Mary Anne has temper tantrums, at least once a week. During the tantrums, Mary Anne bangs her head and bites herself. She also does not seem to tolerate heat and does not appear to sweat normally. Her attention and activity level were reported to be within normal limits.

Her physical examination revealed several remarkable findings including slightly depressed nasal tip, mild facial hypotonia, abnormal lung sounds, enlarged tonsils, and bilateral short fifth fingers. Her speech and language skills were reported to be delayed. Mary Anne's foster parents reported that they would only be able to keep Mary Anne for an additional twelve months. At the end of that time, they will be moving out of state. The social worker hopes to reunite Mary Anne with her maternal grandmother.

Questions

- What referrals would you make and why?
- Which tests would you include in your assessment protocol for speech and language skills?
- How would you plan for Mary Ann's reunion with her family?

CASE FOUR

Kyle is a one-month-old male referred to the Special Children's Clinic because of drug exposure in utero. Reportedly, Kyle visually tracts objects and people, reacts to sounds, and gives clear communicative cues. Kyle's birth mother reportedly smoked cigarettes during her pregnancy with Kyle but denies drug and alcohol use. Kyle was born full term at home and weighed six pounds, nine ounces. He was taken to the University Medical Center's nursery after birth. Mom's toxicology screen was positive for cocaine and methamphetamines. Kyle presented with jaundice and received phototherapy.

At one month, Kyle lives with a foster family. He presented to the doctor with a cold, weakness in the upper right extremity, and increased muscle tone in trunk and lower extremities. His immunization status is unknown. The results of the Denver Developmental Screening II suggest that Kyle presents with delays in personal–social skills, gross motor skills, and language skills. Fine motor skills were judged to represent a caution.

Social services reported that mom is in rehabilitation and is expected to make good progress. If she is able to make significant progress, she will be able to return to her position as a department store manager. Social services hopes to reunite Kyle with his mother at some point. Kyle has two brothers living in two different foster care placements. One is seven and the other is three years old. The social worker hopes that all can be reunited soon.

Questions

- What recommendations would you make for stimulating the development of oral–motor skills?
- What plan would you present for language stimulation?
- Would you make additional referrals? Why or why not?

SUMMARY

As frequently reported in the literature, the case studies presented demonstrate that the clinical presentations of children having a history of substance abuse and HIV vary greatly. Many children from this special population exhibit the characteristics ascribed to the typically developing child. Others present with physical and social characteristics that distinguish them from typically developing children. For example, some may present with medical fragility. Still others display varying types and degrees of learning disabilities. Larsen (1998), in her text, describes the medical, physical, and social aspects of pediatric HIV. She points out that children with HIV typically experience a host of medically related problems. Some of the problems may include chronic respiratory and pulmonary disease, acquired microcephaly, failure to thrive, recurrent bacterial pneumonia or infections, recurrent otitis media, sinusitis, mastoiditis, chronic oral candidiasis, esophagistis, dysphagia, odynophagia, enlarged liver and spleen, enlarged lymph nodes, and/or encephalopathy. Larsen cites numerous studies (Armstrong, Seidel, and Swales, 1993; Belman, 1992; Pressman, 1992; Seidel, 1991) suggesting that school-age children with pediatric HIV sometimes exhibit a variety of motor, speech, language, hearing, and cognitive deficits. Attention deficit disorder and behavioral problems may also complicate the therapeutic and educational process for children living with HIV.

In addition, factors such as, poor prenatal care, prematurity, low birth weight, mothers who are ill because of HIV infection often occur with this population. Children with prenatal exposure to substance abuse, whether co-occurring with HIV or not, have been reported to experience loss of state control, irritability, attention deficit disorder, learning disabilities, and frequent middle ear infections (Larsen, 1998).

The case studies provided illustrate the complex case histories often associated with this population. Some children spend the first weeks of life in the neonatal care unit with the staff of nurses and doctors acting as primary caregivers. Some children struggling with substance abuse and HIV go home with birth families. Some children will probably live in several different foster homes during their childhood. Some children in foster care may live in as many as ten different foster homes before receiving emancipation at the age of eighteen. The cases illustrate how the clinicians gathered information about the life and lifestyle of the children and their families whenever and however possible. We hope that you use this historical data to develop your recommendations for intervention.

REFERENCES

Armstrong, F., Seidal, J., and T. Swales (1993). Pediatric HIV Infection: A Neuropsychological and Educational Challenge. *Journal of Learning Disabilities.* 26, 92-103.

Belman, A. (1992). Acquired Immunodeficiency Syndrome and the Child's Central Nervous System. *Pediatric Clinics of North America.* 39, 691-714.

Larsen, C. (1998). *HIV-1 and Communication Disorders: What Speech and Hearing Professionals Need to Know.* San Diego: Singular Publishing Group. Inc.

Pressman, H. (1992). Communication Disorders and Dysphagia in Pediatric AIDS. *ASHA.* 34, 45-47.

Seidel, J. (1991). The Development of a Comprehensive Pediatric HIV Developmental Service Program. In: A. Rudigier, ed. *Technical Report on Developmental Disabilities and HIV Infection* (no. 7), 1-4. Silver Spring, MD: American Association of Affiliated Programs.

Index

Page numbers followed by the letter "e" indicate exhibits; those followed by the letter "t" indicate tables.

HIV, Substance Abuse, and Communication Disorders in Children
© 2007 by The Haworth Press, Inc. All rights reserved.
doi:10.1300/5438_11

T - #0600 - 101024 - C0 - 212/152/7 - PB - 9780789027122 - Gloss Lamination